How To Dine Like The Devil and Feel Like a Saint: Good-bye to Guilty Eating

Luc De Schepper

MD., Ph.D. Lic.Ac., C.Hom., D.I. Hom.

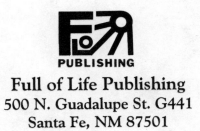

PUBLISHING

Full of Life Publishing
500 N. Guadalupe St. G441
Santa Fe, NM 87501

From the same author:

"Acupuncture for the Practitioner, " 1985

"Candida, the Causes, the Symptoms, the Cure," 1986

"Peak Immunity," 1989

"Full of Life," 1991

"Human Condition: Critical," 1993

1 st. printing

Library of Congress Catalog Card number: 93-70914

ISBN 0-94-2501-01-2

Printed in the United States of America by Community Press, Provo, UTAH

The information in this book is not intended as medical advice. Its intention is solely informational and educational. It is assumed that the reader will consult a medical or health professional should the need for one be warranted.

Full of Life Publishing, Santa Fe, NM 87501

Dedicated to my wife Yolanda and Mom Betty

ACKNOWLEDGMENTS

I want to thank my mother-in-law for the many recipes she brought to this book. Many thanks go to my dear wife, Yolanda, for the drawings, the cover and the photographs. I am grateful for the dedicated formatting work of my friend Ken DeSure, D.C.. Mr. Kampion deserves my respect for proofreading this book. And thanks to all my patients who have wanted this book and pushed me to completing it. May better health be the result!

Luc De Schepper M.D., Ph.D., Lic.Ac., C.Hom., D.I.Hom.
500 North Guadalupe Street, Suite G441
Santa Fe, NM 87501

New Practice address
Luc De Schepper M.D.
16 W. River Rd
Rumson, NJ 07760
Tel. 908-842-9889

Full of Life Publishing
500 N. Guadalupe St
G441
Santa Fe, NM 87501
USA
FAX 505-982-4011

Cover by Yolanda De Schepper

Table of Contents

You want to keep this feeling
Supplements to keep your energy

INTRODUCTION

"The cure of many diseases is unknown to the physicians of Hellas, because they are ignorant of the whole, which ought to be studied also; for the part can never be well unless the whole is well.... This is the great error of our day in the treatment of the human body, that the physicians separate the soul from the body."

These words of wisdom come down to us from the Greek philosopher, Plato. Perhaps the most astonishing aspect of its message, delivered in 427 BC., is that it could have been said by any modern day philosopher. Over the intervening millennia, medical practitioners have continued to dissect and treat the human body as if its parts somehow operated independently of one another. As for the emotions and the soul at the core of our humanity, they are relegated to the care of a completely different breed of healer.

During the 1990s the world will face a staggering array of health problems, most of which will defy easy solutions. New illnesses and complications will test the ingenuity of scientists, doctors, and patients alike. Paradoxically, however, there is some cause for hope. Among the population there is growing recognition that many of our most serious maladies are self-inflicted, the result of too much alcohol, too much food, too many drugs, cigarettes, and indiscriminate sex.

Samuel Hahnemann, the founder of homeopathic medicine and, in my eyes, a true medical genius, proclaimed in his *Organon of the Healing Art* (1810):

"those diseases are inappropriately named chronic which persons incur who expose themselves continually to avoidable noxious influences, who are in the habit of indulging in injurious liquors, or aliments... These states of health, which persons bring upon themselves disappear spontaneously, under an improved mode of living, and they cannot be called chronic diseases."

Westerners generally regard a person as being well so long as she or he is not declared sick. However, almost always, by the time a disease is detected by a person or a doctor, it has already progressed a long way. At that point, the real causes are usually in the relatively distant past, where some breach of harmony and state of lowered resistance invited viruses and microbes to gain the upper hand.

Ultimately, we all need to think in terms of promoting well-being and preventing illness, rather than waiting for the onset of disease to mount a defense. For some practitioners this has always been the goal. And, indeed, we have seen a recent renaissance in this viewpoint. Clearly, the attuned physician of the '90s must also serve as a wellness advisor and a lifestyle expert.

Such a position is demanded by the state of conventional modern medicine. For all the technological miracles it is able to perform, many medical experts have become skeptical of the proliferation of expensive high-tech treatments. Many of these modalities seem to be randomly allowed and practiced in different states, and there are frightening implications when the type of therapy one is allowed to receive in one state can be more aggressive than in another.

Even more astonishing than significant differences in treatment patterns is the fact that those who receive less radical therapies often do better than those treated more "aggressively." Two hundred years ago, Hahnemann's ideal treatment was to find the "most gentle treatment, the treatment that would disturb the Vital Energy the least."

Despite all of our technological advances, you might be surprised to learn that most doctors' response to patient disease is based more on intuition than on scientifically-valid test results. Surging health care costs (and, therefore, a lack of health insurance for many patients) is beginning to change all that.

Full of Life

If we were to follow Plato's advise, each person would become an active participant in her or his own health plan. My book *Full of Life* teaches each of us how to discover the time bombs in our bodies and how to deactivate them before they can do their worst damage. Patients have to realize that recognizing the "triggering factors of illness," as they are described in *Full of Life*, is vital to the success of any treatment plan ultimately decided upon.

Full of Life extensively discusses the various groups of triggering factors that you, as a diligent Sherlock Holmes, must uncover as the culprits on your way to solving the mystery of your own well-being. Of all these culprits, the one we have the most control over is our diet. I recently read that Julia Child laments the spreading fear of consuming butter, cream, saturated fats, and cholesterol.

In my opinion, she doesn't know the half of it. There is also plenty of justified anxiety concerning the abundance of hormones, pesticides, coloring substances, toxins, and other additives--all in one dish--that threaten to ruin more than just our appetites.

The Age of the Quick Fix

What is life, and what should be done with our individual piece of it? Do we really behave as if we want to enjoy rewarding, decent lives filled with good humor and good health? Do we understand the connectedness--the holism--of all things? Or do we, too, see the brain as separate from the spine, the heart separate from the soul? Do we take responsibility for ourselves, understanding that we reap what we sow, or do we blame society for not providing the bounties we think should rightfully be ours?

At times our childish mentality can spawn unrealistic expectations of life and the world around us. Specifically, we are increasingly addicted to the quick, the painless, and the convenient.

Perhaps the best example of our appetite for quick solutions can be seen in our response to the weight crisis. Today, a record-breaking 30 million Americans are <u>at least</u> 20 percent overweight, this according to the American Medical Association. At any given moment 40 percent of all American adults are involved in some type of weight-loss plan. According to the best estimates, however, barely five percent of these dieters will be able to maintain their weight loss permanently.

Losing weight is a big business, and growing. Yet the $33,000,000,000 (that's billions) Americans spend annually to shed pounds bring poor and sometimes life-threatening results. For example, there is a worrisome trend away from exercise and toward so-called "fast" diets, which ignore nutritional safety. Liquid diets have become a crash course for millions. "Slim" companies are hawked and endorsed by high-profile celebrities whose weight losses mean big gains for the shake-makers. In fact, in just one year, 20 million Americans spend almost $1 billion on medically-supervised and over-the-counter liquid-diet products. And still, we don't really know if this self-induced liquid-formula starvation is safe; curiously, there is a paucity of governmental regulation to reduce the users' risk. Moreover, users often go on binges, relying on the "miracle" liquid to repair the damage. As a result, liquid dieters haven't really done anything to improve their eating habits and, unless they drink the powder for the rest of their lives, will inevitably regain the weight.

The craze for miracle diets is supported and demonstrated on the magazine racks at the check-out lanes of your local market. You can't miss those wonderful promises on the covers: "Lose 30 pounds in 30 days!" I have always suspected that a good chunk of those 30 pounds must come from brain cell attrition. Otherwise, how could people be so gullible as to believe that miracle diets work? After all, there is a new one hitting the bookstores every month, but the problem hasn't gone away, has it?

So, give up the quest for your "miracle diet." **There isn't one!**

Losing weight requires commitment and a willingness to be responsible, make changes, and take risks. Only a long-term maintenance weight-loss program (often designed by the patient herself) will make a lasting difference. On the other hand, the yo-yo dieters, are caught up in the gain-lose-gain pattern because they view their succession of diets as harsh, restrictive, and dull. It's no wonder they go back to overeating!

A Word on Motivation

Why did I write this book?

As a physician trained in traditional Western medicine as well as Eastern and alternative medicines (acupuncture, homeopathy, and supplement therapy), I am in a good position to compare the efficacy of different approaches. Western medicine views our health problems as an ongoing war against disease. It uses toxic chemicals and a surgical knife to win the battle. It is a barbaric form of medicine that has been refined and enhanced through technology, but its essential philosophy (man versus nature) remains unchanged.

As a vitalist and an holistic practitioner, I prefer to promote health and wellness, not disease. True, radiation and chemotherapies kill cancer cells, but they also simultaneously decrease the patient's <u>vital energy</u>; this is expressed through hairloss, chronic diarrhea, opportunistic infections, and so on.

As a Western doctor, I am familiar with the attitude that we can control the body, that as physicians we are ordained to be commanders over <u>your</u> body. But as an holistic doctor, I ask: how much more sense does it make for me to become the teacher of my patients? This is the better way, I know. If I try to command you, or even if you try to command yourself, we will only generate resistance. We will, in the end, only strengthen that which we set out to weaken. Only a true understanding of the interrelationships of all things can bring about permanent change.

I want to educate you because I believe that health does not come necessarily from the treatment itself, but from the healing abilities <u>within you</u>. An effective remedy is one that supports and strengthens the patient's own healing abilities. We need to become more aware of the factors that <u>preserve</u> health, not only with the agents of disease. When we understand the factors that work synergistic with the preservation of our Vital Energy, we come to understand our ultimate responsibility for our own health.

When this happens, we become our own health-care professional; we're in the business of preventive medicine.

This is where my diet book comes in. I am offering you, the reader, a valuable tool, one that will serve as a starting point on your path to become <u>full of life</u>. This cookbook is not about improving strength and fitness, per se; it's designed for anyone who wants to prevent the breach of balance that leads one down the path to illness. This is a healing book, too, in the sense that it provides you, the reader, with a clear pathway to positive action and lasting results.

No matter the state of your health, this cookbook will help you reach your next level of energy. Reading it and working with its principles and menus, you will soon realize that this approach is different than anything else out there. In addition to a very well-balanced, day-by-day recipe plan for a six-week period, this book describes the daily bodily changes each person will undergo. These body changes, sometimes perceived as very uncomfortable, can be mitigated with a variety of supplements and homeopathic remedies. These are outlined for each step of the diet. This book also teaches the reader to recognize objective symptoms, thus enabling the patient to recognize the unfolding of the process.

Above all, this is an extremely positive book. I am not interested in reciting a litany of horror stories. In fact, I believe that eating is one of life's greatest pleasures. But to keep the pleasure from leading us toward some future nightmare, we must learn to eat well and eat wisely. And remember: food is not the only hazard in our lives that we have control over; we also can limit the dangers of smoking, alcohol and drug consumption, unsafe working conditions, and lack of exercise.

We just have to understand how it all fits together: **Life, Joy, Love.**

Start Here, Start Now

We all know the different types of eaters. There are the so-called Health Nuts, who limit their intake of animal fats, eating only "organically-grown" foods, plenty of vegetables, grains, and fruits while avoiding all sugar and additives. At the opposite extreme is the meat-and-potato consumer, whose idea of a good meal includes sizable portions of sausage, bacon, ham, hot dogs, and a range of high-cholesterol foods at every opportunity.

Vegan or beef-lover, there are further categories of eaters, such as the "meal skippers," who will skip breakfast and sometimes lunch to keep last night's late snacking from increasing their waist size. Then, there are the "hurried eaters," who are inclined to eat frozen prepared meals, snack foods, soft drinks, and the road delicate cuisine of our modern fast-food restaurants.

No matter what type of eater you are, by following the guidelines in this book you will enjoy healthier dining and make some significant improvement in your life. Because, who doesn't want to be full of life, from the morning on?

The <u>Full of Life</u> program is divided into three phases. I have provided each of these stages with an ample smorgasbord of delicious recipes.

1) <u>Cleansing Phase</u>: Lasting four weeks, this crucial period is out-lined along with a treasure throve of information on how to get yourself through the most uncomfortable symptoms. However, you will never, in fact, feel "deprived" since the recipes are delicious and easy to prepare.

2) <u>Stabilization Phase</u>: During the next two weeks, helpful supplements and homeopathic remedies support your body in its changes and make the ongoing transition easier.

3) <u>Full-of-Life Phase</u>: The goal and the reward all in one, I have outlined how you will feel at this point, what supplements you will need to maintain this energetic stage, and how to be alert for symptoms of decreased health and possible return to previous stages.

In this book, I have also taken into account our different lifestyles. Perhaps you have business-dinner obligations or you have trouble handling family members who are "food pushers." The chapter, "*Life on the Road,*" tells you how to navigate your ship of health through these minefields without either weakening or becoming overly frustrated.

Modern times have indeed created a real need for fast, healthy prepared meals. After a hard days' work, you may well not have the energy nor the desire to spend another two hours in your kitchen. The chapter, "*Cooking in the Fast Lane,*" offers valuable, proven tips and recipes that will carry you through those hard times while still eliciting admiring looks and appreciative words from family and friends.

And don't worry. I have <u>not</u> forgotten those special times of the year. Holidays, birthdays, and special occasions demand a more fanciful and elaborate menu. The chapter, "*It's Party Time,*" offers a range of wonderful ideas for entertaining family and guests without threat of being accused of preparing something that is too dull.

CHAPTER ONE

EAT YOUR WAY TO PEAK IMMUNITY: SEVEN PRINCIPLES OF HEALTHY EATING

"Temporary diets don't work. Basic principles of good nutrition, followed for a lifetime, do."

Principle #1: Make the Decision to Eat Well

Americans are obsessed with losing weight. Most bookstores have a few shelves -- or a whole section -- filled with the newest books on diet and weight loss. Yet, despite the proliferation of commercial weight-loss centers and a hoard of diet formulas, most people find themselves in the yo-yo syndrome -- losing several pounds, only to gain them back when once the normal pattern of eating is restored. And as the weight cycling increases (on and off, on and off), so does the risk of heart disease. These patients, quite justifiably, feel very restricted and frustrated.

We all know that overeating is not good. The media tell us so; the American Heart Association and American Cancer Society do too. Why, then, is it so hard for people to make real changes in their eating patterns?

Diets are restrictive, and when people feel deprived, they can't -- and won't -- maintain a routine that continues this deprivation. Although the trend is beginning to change, fad and commercial diets generally put too much emphasis on limiting calories and not enough on good nutrition.

To be successful and to truly help people, an eating plan needs to take into consideration the whole person. "Dieters" should be encouraged to examine all the aspects of their lives, not just how many calories they're taking in. We must learn to identify the factors that trigger our overeating. We need to learn how to use their leisure time, how to handle job and relationship stress, how to develop regular exercise habits. In support groups like Overeaters Anonymous (OA), people learn how to pinpoint the triggers for their overeating. When they can learn to deal with them, healthy, nutritious eating will follow.

Why We Overeat

We don't eat merely to satisfy our physical hunger. The act of eating is loaded with social and emotional implications. This is not new, of course. Throughout history, human beings have used meals as a stage for celebration and an occasion to mark important cultural and personal events. But consuming food to satisfy our emotional hunger is a destructive mixing of two very different worlds.

There are several types of "emotional eater." The most common includes those who eat to escape depression. For them, food provides a great comfort. When family or friends are critical of us or disappoint us, relief through food is generally the most available antidote. The pattern may have started with our parents, but it is effectively reinforced by the media. When it's cold and rainy outside, and you had a hard day at school, what's more comforting than coming home to homebaked cookies and milk? After a brutal day at the office, television and snacks re-establishes a sense of well-being.

The unfortunate reality, however, is that the relief we gain from food is short-lived. To be effective, we have to keep feeding that emotional appetite. Even so, the foods we eat may give us a momentary "high," but the letdown is worse, adding extra pounds and guilt to the original depression.

Eating the Wrong Foods

Perhaps you don't eat too much. Some of us who are quite slim have a different problem: eating the wrong foods. We all know that "junk food" is bad for us, but it's absurdly difficult to switch to good food. Why is this?

Most people think of "health food" as tasteless, colorless, and crudely textured. This is a misconception. In fact, health food (or whole food) suffers from a bad rap. We perceive these foods as bland or strange because our taste buds (and emotional appetites) have been conditioned and programmed to expect the salt-fat-sugar flavors. It is possible to retrain and reprogram your taste buds, however.

Eliminate sugar from your diet for a period of time, and then try one of your favorite candy bars. It might not seem the treat you thought it would be; at the very least you will become aware of its extraordinarily excessive sweetness. The same is true of salty foods. Once you become accustomed to foods that are either unsalted or lightly salted, you will immediately notice the overuse of salt in restaurant and frozen foods.

Food Controversies

Perhaps you're already eating healthy food. But even then you run into another little problem: health professionals don't agree on what constitutes a healthy diet. The cholesterol controversy has been a prime example. Years ago, people ate a lot of fish, eggs, and meat. Then eggs and fish fell into disgrace in favor of the Omega-6 fats of deep-fried foods. But after a 1984 Harvard Medical School study of the eating habits of Eskimos, fish such as salmon and halibut (which contain Omega-3 fats) were again recommended.

One of the more recent food controversies, generating a wave of consumer confusion, has been over the benefits of oat bran. The "cholesterol-lowering effect of oats" got especially high marks, even in highly respected medical journals such as The Lancet (footnote 1), a British medical journal, and the American Journal of Clinical Nutrition (footnote 2). Then a 1990 study, published in the New England Journal of Medicine, concluded that oat bran was no better than plain white flour when it came to lowering cholesterol levels. This put a damper on oat sales; however, only 20 people (all with relatively low cholesterol levels) participated in the study.

Such controversies do not instill confidence in consumers. One might conclude, "Why bother? If the experts can't make up their minds, we might as well eat Twinkies™, chocolate bars, and potato chips today, because we can expect that some expert might decide that these are healthy tomorrow."

There is another, prominent, source of confusion in the world of nutrition. Although many people today know more about the link between diet and disease than the typical physician did in the 1970s, much of the awareness comes from food advertising, not from health professionals. This has contributed to continuing confusion over the specifics of the diet-health link. For instance, in part due to abundant advertising and packaging claims, most people still do not understand the difference between cholesterol and saturated fat in food.

In fact, when choosing foods that are less damaging to your heart, you should examine the saturated fat rather than the cholesterol content. Polyunsaturated oils such as corn, sunflower, and safflower are healthful, so long as they are consumed in moderate quantities. Mono-unsaturates, such as almond, olive, avocado, and walnut oil, are the most healthful.

What Is Organic?

In relation to the universe of the US. food market, organic means "grown without the introduction of chemical pesticides and chemicals." Since the alar-tainted apple scare of '89 and the ongoing threat posed by grapes loaded with pesticides, America's interest in chemical-free food has exploded. After years of struggling for recognition and acceptance, the organic food industry is experiencing a boom in popularity. Organically-grown food is now considered mainstream. More growers are experimenting with this environmentally-sensitive approach; extensive research is seeking alternatives to conventional farming with its reliance upon chemicals to combat mold and soil quality problems.

A farm must be chemical free for at least three years before its produce can truly be termed organic, as defined by most organic certification programs, such as CCOF (California Certified Organic Farmers), the OGBA (Organic Growers and Buyers Association of Minnesota), NOFA (National Organic Farmers Association of New York), and the Texas and Washington State programs. Anything less than that is <u>not</u> acceptable.

But how do you know for sure at the market? Is food labeled "organic" really what it says? And according to whom? To the average customer, organically-grown tomatoes might look suspiciously like the "commercial" tomato selling for half the price in the store down the street. In actuality, to be completely sure that you're getting truly organic food, you'd have to grow it yourself. That's no small feat, given our crowded time schedules and the limited availability of land. The most practical approach is to educate yourself and to ask questions of your grocer. If there is no certification label on the box, ask your grocer to produce it.

Make no mistake about it, it takes a considerable effort to maintain a healthful diet in this age of packaged and processed food products. The road to full-of-life energy will take you into new markets, new books, and a whole new world of like-minded individuals who are trying to do their best to be their best.

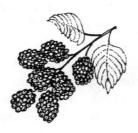

1. DeGroot, A.P., et al. "Cholesterol-lowering Effects of Rolled Oats." Lancet, vol. 2 (1963), pp. 303-4.
2. Kirby, R. W. et al. "Oat-Bran Intake Selectively Lowers Serum Low-Density Lipoprotein Cholesterol Concentrations of Hypercholesterolemic Men." American Journal of Clinical Nutrition, vol. 34 (1981), pp. 824-8.

Principle #2: Avoid the Diet Traps!

No matter what eating plan you ultimately choose, some additional elements have to be present if you're going to succeed.

Flexibility
Does your selected plan:

- Allow you to eat away from home? (Eating out could become increasingly difficult if restaurants don't change the way they do things.)
- Allow you to eat foods you like and give you healthy and tasty recipes for newly introduced foods?
- Offer a regimen low in sugar and fats but high in complex carbohydrates and protein?
- Encourage exercise and teach new eating habits, mostly through behavior-modification techniques?
- Achieve these goals safely and inexpensively?
- Promise long-lasting change and not a quick fix?

If you answered "no" to just one of the questions above, chances are that the food plan will let you down in the long run. To be successful, you'll need real-world flexibility in your new eating plan. Keep searching.

Common Sense Rules

Once you have found a diet program that will work for you, the following common sense rules will be applicable. Whether you are being treated for an immune-suppressed condition or are simply trying to boost your immune system, you will be given specific eating guidelines by your holistic doctor. And at the end of this chapter, sample food lists are provided.

- Chew food thoroughly (20 times for each mouthful). Digestion begins in the mouth with the enzymes in your saliva. Most immune-suppressed conditions (Chronic Fatigue and Immune Dysfunction Syndrome or CFIDS) have some relation to malabsorption. In this syndrome, digestion is so poor that the body's cells are unable to draw nutrients from the food; this leads to states of toxicity, obesity, and sluggishness.

• Drink liquids <u>between</u> meals, not <u>with</u> meals. Drinking liquids during meals dilutes digestive juices.

• Eat only in the dining room and with the rest of your family if possible. Dinner must again become a feast at which manners are observed and joys are shared.

• Don't skip meals. Many people think they are making the right move by skipping breakfast and sometimes lunch as well. The result is a lazy digestive system that lacks the continuous stimulus provided by food intake. "Night-eating syndrome" leads to burning fewer calories. Breakfast is especially easy to omit, but the word "breakfast" should be a reminder that you are "breaking the fast" of the previous night.

• When emotionally upset, eat less. Digestive chemistry is altered with stress, inhibiting complete digestion. In reality, most people will stuff themselves when upset, drawing them into a spiraling cycle of depression and physical discomfort.

• Keep a brief food-related-symptoms journal for everything you eat or drink to learn more about how specific foods affect your disposition and health. Record foods eaten and subsequent reactions over a period of time, then use the diary to identify problem foods.

• Avoid watching TV, listening to radio, or reading while eating. These activities will distract you from focusing on chewing thoroughly and prevent you from maintaining the relaxed mental state which assists digestion and nutrient absorption.

• Read labels and ingredients on boxed, canned, and packaged foods.

• When dining out, ask questions about the ingredients used in preparing your food. Be prepared to be assertive. Some waiters may not bother to communicate your small wishes to the kitchen. When you say, "I can't have any sugar, MSG, soy sauce, or preservatives," they may think, "It's only another health nut making my job difficult." Often wait persons think they can ignore such requests and you won't even notice. Yet a person suffering from Candida, CFIDS, or other malabsorption syndromes can react severely to any number of substances. I know of one CFIDS patient who gets the waiter's attention by telling him that the last time she ingested MSG, the restaurant had to send her to the hospital! You may not feel comfortable being this dramatic, but the server is more likely to get the message that your small request is a critical one. Another idea: Some people prepare small cards itemizing the foods they must avoid and present one to their waiter at the appropriate time. This spares them a recitation and ensures that the waiter won't "forget."

• Eat only when you're hungry. The average person eats for many reasons, most of them suspect -- because it is six o'clock, because they're upset, because they happen to be with friends and food is a wonderful form of communication and entertainment, to have something to do.

• A longer space between meals enables the digestive system to recuperate. Enzymes can be manufactured in sufficient quantities to ensure effective digestion of the next meal. Most of us would do well eating only breakfast and dinner, with nothing between. Except for our habits, we'd perfectly happy.

• Stop blaming someone or something else. You've probably most of the common excuses (or maybe you've even used a few yourself!): "My husband doesn't support my efforts to lose weight," "I had all that food in my refrigerator and I couldn't let it spoil," or the all-time favorite, "I don't have time to shop for this health food and I certainly don't have the time to prepare it." (In reality, it doesn't take much more time to prepare a healthy meal than junk food.) Another favorite target of blame is the doctor who prescribed whatever "stupid diet" you're on that "doesn't allow me to eat anything."

• Last of all, remember: there are no quick fixes, only permanent ones brought about through the modification of our behavior.

By incorporating these common sense rules into any eating plan, you'll be laying the groundwork for your own success. Realize, too, that changing your eating patterns is an ongoing process; it pays to be patient and forgiving with yourself. Being too hard on yourself is not only a sure way to feel worse, it also sets up a resistant "no!" in you that dooms even the most sincere efforts to failure.

Another thought: many people prefer to change their eating habits in stages rather than all at once. If you feel the need to eliminate only the worst elements of your diet at first, before proceeding to the complete peak-immunity diet, then do so. The ultimate responsibility for our eating habits and our health, is ours and ours alone. One aspect of the wisdom of successful change is in pacing ourselves; we need to push our limits, not go beyond them.

Principle #3: Health Begins With Proper Food Combining

Often a patient will ask me, "Why am I not losing weight? Why am I still bloated and uncomfortable after eating, even when eating only the good foods? I'm eating less than my friend who has weird eating habits, yet he never has a weight problem and seems always to have plenty of energy."

The "weird eating habits" mentioned in such reports are often actually references to individuals who practice <u>food combining</u>. While allowed-food lists and calorie counts are most commonly stressed in a dietary plan, food combining is not. This is a great mistake!

Food combining is a practice based on the nutritional discovery that certain combinations of food are digested with greater efficiency than others. The digestion of food consumes more energy than any other function of the human body. After lunch, for instance, increased blood circulation to the digestive system can deplete the brain's oxygen, making you sleepy in the early afternoon. However, for all the body's efforts, only food that is completely broken down by our enzymes will actually be absorbed by the blood and transferred to our cells. Combining food properly maximizes the efficiency of the digestive process causing it to require less energy while extracting more benefit from the food. It is especially important that CFIDS patients adhere to food combining rules, since these people suffer from malabsorption (caused by yeast overgrowth or the presence of parasites).

Let's take a typical American lunch or dinner: a baked potato, a steak, vegetables, followed by a fruit dessert. Consider what happens during this meal. The steak requires an acid digestive juice (hydrochloric acid) to break it down. But the baked potato, eaten during the same meal, requires an alkaline one. It does not take a scientific genius to predict that acid and alkaline digestive enzymes will neutralize each other; this signals the body to produce more juices, since digestion is incomplete. But the newly produced juices are again neutralized. In the meantime, having been held too long in the stomach, the meat has begun to putrefy and the potato has had time to ferment, causing bloating, gas, and discomfort. To make matters worse, such repetitive efforts by the digestive system to do its job can lead ultimately to its exhaustion. When this happens, the hardy individual who proudly ate anything and everything (and in any combination) suddenly finds allergic-like reactions setting in.

To make matters worse, many people top their meal off with a "healthy" fruit desert. This compounds the problem. Fruit can be absorbed by the body directly, so the long digestive process is bypassed. Indeed, watermelon, apples, oranges, cantaloupe, grapefruit, peaches, and prunes pass through the stomach in less than an hour, compared to the two hours or more required by other foods. If you eat fruits for dessert, they will be held in your stomach longer than they should. This creates even more fermentation and putrefaction, requiring an even larger expenditure of energy to push the mass into the small intestine. Once there, another 24 hours are required for the food to complete its journey through the intestinal tract. Still surprised that you feel bloated, gassy, seven months pregnant, and dead tired at two o'clock in the afternoon? With your digestion in such a state, it's surprising your brain can work at all!

To modify your current diet to create proper food combinations, you must remember that different foods require different lengths of time (and different enzymes) to be broken down. Here are some basic rules-of-thumb to help in planning your menus:

• Fatty foods are the most difficult for the body to digest. Fried foods, gravies, rich sauces, pastries, shrimp, ham, pork, and bacon may require up to five hours for digestive breakdown into smaller compounds. Can you imagine what havoc these goodies create in your stomach when they're eaten with veggies and fruit?

• For proper digestion, "one protein at a time" is a golden rule. Different proteins require different enzymes for digestion, so don't combine cheese, for example, with chicken. In many cases, the different digestive enzymes required by different proteins may cancel each other out.

• Melons should always be eaten alone. They digest so easily that they proceed through the stomach faster than any other fruit. Combining melon even with other fruits, such as apples and pears, will hold up its digestion long enough to cause extensive fermentation.

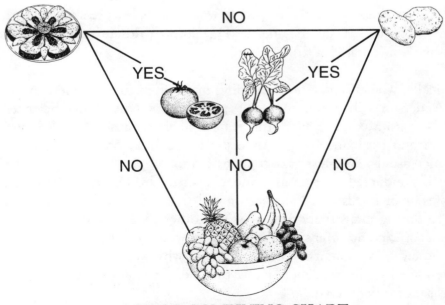

FOOD COMBINING CHART

Principle #4: You Crave Your Own Personal Poison

Anyone who suffers from candidiasis and/or CFIDS knows that cravings can rule their life. There is an irresistible urge, a <u>driven</u> feeling within the body, to consume particular foods. What do these cravings mean? Do they fulfill certain basic physiological needs? And how can you cope with them when they happen to you?

<u>Causes of the Cravings</u>

In an article entitled "Does Your Body Know What It Needs? Cravings" (Good Health Magazine, New York Times, September 27, 1987), various opinions are expressed on the subject:

• "There is no physiological reason to explain these cravings" (Dr. Richard Mattes of the Monell Chemical Center in Philadelphia, PA);

• "These foods are craved because their consumption will either satisfy a nutritional deficiency or, particularly with carbohydrate cravings [attention Candidiasis-sufferers!], serve as a form of self-medication to counteract depression" (Dr. Judith Wurtman, Biochemist at the Massachusetts Institute of Technology, Boston);

• "Carbohydrate cravings are linked to people with seasonal depressions and, therefore, what they crave is actually what they need" (Dr. Norman Rosenthal, psychiatrist at the National Institute of Mental Health).

Statistically, women report food cravings more often than do men. According to Dr. Harvey Anderson, Chairman of the Department of Nutritional Sciences at the University of Toronto Medical School, this is most likely because of food desires related to menstruation and pregnancy. Dr. Anderson found that, on average, carbohydrate consumption increases by 30% just prior to menstruation.

Research conducted at Kansas State University by Dr. Katharina Grunewald, Associate Professor of Foods and Nutrition, found that most women in a study craved chocolate more during menstruation than at any other time of the month. However, cravings for popcorn, potato chips, and hamburgers were not affected by the menstrual cycle. Dr. Grunewald comments: "We don't know why women crave more chocolate during the menstrual cycle, we simply know they do. It may be that they want to do something pleasant for themselves."

In Chapter two of my book, *Full of Life*, you will find a different explanation for food cravings. The Chinese believe that when we crave a certain taste (sweet, salty, spicy), the organ associated with that taste is suffering. The spleen-pancreas, for instance, is suffering when we crave sweets and other carbohydrates (CBH). And, to some extent, it is true that their consumption will satisfy a nutritional deficiency. Moderate amounts of CBH (extreme cases of Candida/CFIDS will not tolerate this at all) and sweets <u>will</u> strengthen the spleen-pancreas. However, when patients experience cravings, they are not talking in terms of "moderate amounts." Usually the patient will be drawn to a roller coaster ride of sugar intake and reaction, leading to quite the opposite of the desired balancing effect. Consumption of sugar or CBH will improve a patient's mood for just a very short period of time, perhaps half an hour. Afterwards, inevitably, they are likely to collapse into severe mood swings and depression.

Women with yeast overgrowth often also have more severe PMS and experience very strong cravings for CBH, especially sweets, in the week or so preceding a menstrual period. The reason for this is simple: Progesterone levels increase before the menstrual cycle, leading to increased glycemia (sugar) in the blood. Yeast cells respond by multiplying faster, sensing the presence of increased sugar. So these cravings actually come from the yeast cells themselves. It is actually the craving of the yeast cells that these women experience as their own craving!

What a mistake, then, for such patients to follow the advice of Dr. Rosenthal, who claims that what they crave is actually what they need! As countless candidiasis sufferers will attest, an increased sugar intake at this time will almost certainly lead them toward more extreme mood swings and deeper depression.

<u>Dealing with the Cravings</u>

Since change begins with acceptance, the first step in overcoming our cravings is to recognize them for what they are: signals to warn you to eliminate the food or taste that you're craving. "Easier said than done," you say. Well, there is some help available:

• Acupuncture has certain points that can cut the cravings immediately, even before you make adjustments to your diet. The best points are K3, LI 4 and Li 3.

• Carnitine, an amino acid, taken in tablet form two to three times a day, can reduce your cravings sufficiently to get you past the initial cravings.

• GTF Chromium, which helps regulate the body's sugar-insulin balance, can be very helpful. Taken three times a day before meals, chromium can be helpful in adult-onset diabetes and in controlling the high-and-low blood-sugar fluctuations of hypoglycemia.

• Green Magma(TM): two tablets three times a day before meals.

• Licorice root: One tablet before each meal helps regulate the blood sugar level, stimulates the adrenals.

• Lycopodium or Argentum Nit. (homeopathic medications): 3 pellets, 15 minutes away from meals; repeat as needed. Indication of these homeopathic remedies is determined according to the laws of homeopathy (See: "*Human Condition: Critical*", Full of Life Publishing, Santa Fe, NM). Intense cravings for sweets will be taken into account by the homeopathic physician to find the appropriate homeopathic remedy. Lycopodium and Argentum Nitricum are high on the list of sweet cravings.

The basic idea of Principle #4 is this: recognize a craving for what it is, and then work to curb it. Natural help is available, as you will learn from the food-choice lists later in this chapter. Above all, stay positive! Once you have clearly identified the source of the cravings and begun some behavioral modification, you may find, as many have, that even sweets no longer taste "as good as they used to."

Principle #5: Increase Energy and Avoid Mood Swings

It's a simple but powerful truth: you can feel healthier, more alive, and far less moody simply by selecting the right kinds of foods. In fact, by effectively managing the food you eat you can alleviate a wide range of disturbing symptoms such as insomnia, morning fatigue, depression and mood swings. The Candida/Peak Immunity diet is a high-protein, low-carbohydrate eating plan designed specifically to address your symptoms.

<u>Protein for Energy</u>

If you are suffering from CFIDS, Candidiasis, or a general lack of energy, eating protein in the morning will increase your energy, neutralize the post-lunch doldrums, and stabilize your psychology throughout the day. But don't go right out and eat steak! Not all proteins will produce the same results. The most effective energy boosters will be proteins that are low in fat, such as fish, shellfish, veal, chicken without the skin, and very lean beef. For healthy people who are not suffering from CFIDS or Candidiasis, low-fat milk and low-fat yogurt will have the same beneficial effects.

Carbos for Calm

If your goal includes achieving a calmer, more relaxed state of mind and increased freedom from anxiety and insomnia, carbohydrates can be good allies. There are two types of carbos: the sugars (glucose, sucrose, fructose, and lactose) and the starchy carbohydrates (potatoes, corn, and vegetables).

Food and the Brain

Why will eating more protein boost your energy, while eating more carbohydrates calms you down and sometimes even makes you sleepy? The answer is in the way the chemical machinery of our body works. Small bits of information are transported from one brain cell to another by means of chemical substances, called neurotransmitters. Two classes of such neurotransmitters are manufactured by the brain from the foods we eat: the "alertness" chemicals dopamine and norepinephrine, and the "calming" chemical serotonin. Tyrosine is the amino acid from which dopamine and norepinephrine are produced. Serotonin is produced from its precursor, tryptophan. These two amino acids (tyrosine and tryptophan) enter the brain along with other essential amino acids. Tryptophan is known for its calming effects. Eating foods rich in this amino acid will have a calming effect. The converse is true of the proteins which break down into the amino acid tyrosine; you'll get a "kick" from ingesting foods high in that amino acid.

In order to feel fit throughout the day, you should eat proteins at breakfast and lunch, when you need the energy. Then eat carbohydrates at night with little protein, to ensure a calming effect.

So you see, Principle #5 is simple: It can be more than a matter of luck to feel more energetic and happily avoid mood swings. If you use the information in this book, you can modify your moods and help your suppressed immune system recover from the years of accumulated distress.

Principle #6: Know Your Fats

Now that "total cholesterol," "HDL and LDL," and "saturated fat" have all become household terms, why do people still have problems selecting and preparing foods that reduce their risk of obesity and heart disease? Conflicting messages on food labels may be one reason; ignorance about possible food "time bombs" may be another. You don't need to go back to school to take extensive courses in nutrition and biochemistry. Simply knowing the differences between saturated and non-saturated fats will contribute more to a low cholesterol count than avoiding cholesterol-rich foods altogether.

Simply put, saturated fat is fat which will become solid at room temperature, like butter or bacon grease. HDL or High Density Lipo-proteins are the "good" cholesterol particles. An increase in this HDL will push your total cholesterol up. But no change is needed in this case. Therefore it is important to know your HDL, not just your total cholesterol. Even better, you should always know your "LDL/HDL risk ratio" or "Relative risk of coronary artery disease". This takes into account the different cholesterols. Your local American Heart Association office is a good source of free booklets and pamphlets on eating for a healthy heart.

Unlikely Sources of Fat

For decades many of our favorite cookies, crackers, and breakfast cereals have been made using highly saturated tropical oils such as lard, coconut oil, and palm oil. As you were munching on your favorite snack, you were also quite possibly clogging your arteries with cholesterol deposits. So why are these saturated fats so commonly used? Because they account for the crunchiness and crispy freshness of our cookies, and these are qualities that the American public insists on. However, all this is changing, due in part to the media attention brought to the dangers of high serum cholesterol levels.

The big food companies have had to make adjustments. They promised to get rid of all these saturated oils and replace them with more healthful, unsaturated oils -- corn or canola, for example. End of the story? Unfortunately, no. Torn between the public's demand for delicious products and the anti-cholesterol movement that's sweeping the country, cookie producers have done the only thing they could: They began saturating the unsaturated fats in a process called "hydrogenation." Now companies could advertise that they were health-consciously using unsaturated fats while still producing our heavenly snacks just the way we like 'em!

What these snack-food makers have forgotten to mention is this: The process of hydrogenating (for instance, soybean oil, probably the most common candidate for hydrogenation) transforms a percentage of this unsaturated oil into saturated fat. That's not the only bad news. Hydrogenation also transforms unsaturated fats into "trans fatty acids" which are stable and solid, and therefore look and act like the dreaded saturated fatty acids. Even so, processors are not required to say anything about the trans-fatty acid content, leaving the gates wide open for the spreading of misinformation on what exactly healthful foods are. As the consumer, you should be aware that the term "partially hydrogenated" is a red flag to your good health. It certainly looks like we can't have our cake and eat it too.

Which to Pick?

What are we to do? Fat is fat, but it wears several different hats. Many people still believe that because they use margarine instead of butter, non-dairy creamers instead of milk and polyunsaturated fats, they are on the path to a healthier diet. Yet, margarine is a synthetic substance, produced by processing vegetable oil, then hydrogenating it to make it solid. This way, an unsaturated fat is transformed into a saturated one. Still, it is better to pick a margarine that has twice as many polyunsaturated fats as saturated ones. For instance, a label indicating five grams of polyunsaturated fat to two grams of saturated fat would indicate a relatively healthy margarine. Non-dairy creamers are still loaded with fats and polyunsaturated fatty acids, which do lower the total cholesterol, but have at the same time the unwanted effect of lowering HDL, our beneficial cholesterol.

What's left, I hear you ask? Follow a few simple rules of thumb and you won't go far wrong:

• Avoid saturated fats -- especially the ones found mainly in cheese, lard and meats -- if at all possible.

• Omit tropical oils, such as coconut, cocoa butter, and palm oil.

• Avoid all hydrogenated food products.

• For you diet, concentrate on the mono-unsaturated fatty acids such as olive, sesame, walnut, cashew, canola, and avocado oils.

• Choose the "extra virgin" olive oil. This term describes the highest quality oil with the best flavor, color, and aroma. It is produced in smaller quantities than other grades and is priced the highest. Oil that does not meet the standard for extra virgin oil is refined to remove impurities, then blended with virgin oil. This blend is labeled "pure" olive oil.

Other necessary changes to reduce fats in your diet include:

• Cook foods by broiling, poaching, or steaming instead of frying.

• Increase (3-5 servings daily) the amount of vegetables, fruits, and beans you eat. These foods will increase your intake of complex carbohydrates, which will in turn help reduce serum cholesterol as well as overall calorie intake.

• Limit cholesterol-rich foods such as egg yolks and organ meats (liver, etc.) (1-2 servings daily or less).

• Avoid: Lard, bacon fat, mayonnaise (except the better ones in health food stores), French fries, fried foods, hamburgers and salami.

Is all this worth the trouble and discomfort? You bet it is! In countries where animal and fat consumption is limited, where the diet is compromised mainly of cereals, grains, and vegetables, the incidence of heart disease, cancer, obesity, and diabetes is rare. We really have met one of the greatest enemies of this century -- and it is fat. Too many people have already dug their graves with their forks; millions of otherwise intelligent people shorten their lives further each day by ingesting fat as if there were no tomorrow.

Principle #6: "When in Doubt, Substitute" is another very direct principle: Recognize the harmful fatty foods and replace them with low-fat alternatives. It's the best guarantee of your future health.

Principle #7: Avoid the Trigger Foods

Now that the basic rules of food choice have been outlined, all you need to know now is what are the foods you absolutely should avoid and which ones can you introduce right away. However, the list of foods to avoid and those that are good to eat is not cast in stone.

For CFIDS and Candidiasis patients, it's best to adhere strictly to this food list until you have a real sense of increased energy. Depending on the other therapeutic approaches you undertake, you could reintroduce foods as soon as five weeks after beginning your Full of Life diet. However, this should be an individual choice; you first have to feel better before you move on to the next phase.

No matter then when you begin to reintroduce foods to your diet, introduce them one food at the time. This will enable you to monitor your reactions to each particular food. If you are introducing three foods at one time, and if you feel poorly one hour after the meal, there would be no way for you to determine which of the three produced reaction.

It is also important to know that some patients react to any fruit intake, no matter what the variety. While this can be a sign of significant yeast overgrowth, I have also seen this sensitivity in patients who were quite free of the infamous fungus. In such cases, the cause was an over-growth of friendly bacteria in the gut by anaerobic bacilli, such as klebsiella, proteus, salmonella and shigella. They ferment glucose very quickly, so the slightest amount of sugar (fruit in this case) leads to a quick fermentation with bloating, gas, abdominal pain, and maldigestion.

In case you suspect bacterial overgrowth or parasite invasion (canine hunger, loose stools alternating with constipation, bloating, weight gain, abdominal pain and fatigue), request that your doctor order a comprehensive stool analysis that will look for each of these bacteria. Proper antibiotic intake often will resolve long-standing mysterious health problems. And don't forget to add your friendly bacteria (Lactobacilli) as long as you are taking these antibiotics.

Forbidden Foods

You might think, at first glance, that some of the following foods belong on the "good" food list. Some of them are on this list because they are fermenting foods (like apples, pears, grapes, wine, beer, champagne, vinegar, tofu, and soy sauce), others because they feed a particular problem in the patient (such as yeast-containing foods like breads, wheat, rye, mushrooms, and dairy products). Others (such as wine) contain sulfites (asthma sufferer beware!) and urethane, which appears naturally during fermentation. Urethane is a chemical long recognized to cause cancer in animals, so this naturally causes concern about its effects on humans.

Even if you are not a CFIDS or Candidiasis patient, you will greatly benefit from omitting the following foods. The majority of the population suffers from poor digestion and malabsorption, and avoiding these foods will greatly enhance the power of anyone's digestive system.

• No breads, including yeast-free wheat and rye breads. Rice, corn, unleavened, and Ponce breads, however, are fine.

• No dairy products, except butter, eggs, goat's milk, goat's cheese, and yogurt. Avoid yogurt from cow's milk.

• No mushrooms, wine, champagne, beer, or anything else that is fermented, such as miso and tofu.

• Avoid certain fruits, especially apples, pears, and grapes, but also watermelon, cantaloupe, oranges, peaches, prunes, dates, or any dried fruits (too much sugar).

• No fruit juices (except the juices of allowed fruits; even then, use them sparingly). Do NOT use fruit juices when fasting!

• No tomato or barbecue sauce (unless you make your own without peppers, sugar, vinegar, syrup).

• No wheat or rye, in crackers, cereal, breads or pasta.

• Avoid salt (use sea salt if necessary).

• No sweeteners, including sugar (absolutely none in any form), aspartame (Nutrasweet™, Sweet-N-Low™,), and molasses.

• No tea or coffee, not even caffeine-free coffee or herbal teas (exceptions are noted below).

• Avoid raw and cold foods (except salads occasionally). Remember, these foods decrease the strength of your digestive organ, the spleen pancreas as outlined in Chapter Two.

• Absolutely no vinegar: in salad dressings, use mustard and mayonnaise.

• No horseradish or peppers.

• No canned foods or fried foods.

• Avoid refrigerated leftovers, especially meat (which can develop mold overnight); freeze any left-overs and heat them up later.

• Avoid ice in drinks.

After reading this list, you might think that there's nothing left in your refrigerator that you CAN eat. Don't despair. Consult the "Good Food List" below.

The Good Food List

Despite the daunting length of the "Forbidden Foods" list above, there are a few things left in the world to eat. Even so, it's a good strategy to rotate even these "good foods" to achieve variety, which will further help to eliminate allergies and sensitivities.

• Some fruits, especially papaya, mango, kiwi, pineapple, banana, honeydew, melon, coconut, guava, grapefruit, and lemons. Eat these fruits in the morning at breakfast; never eat them after meals. About ten percent of patients will not be able to eat fruit at all because of the high fructose content (for instance, in bananas) or because of the high acidity (for instance, in pineapples). CFIDS patients should eat fruit sparingly during the first four weeks of the program.

• Some juices. For instance: water with lemon juice, fresh-squeezed vegetable juices, unsweetened cranberry juice, wheat grass juice, fruit juices of allowed fruits (in moderation), coconut milk.

• Grains: brown rice, wild rice, millet, buckwheat, amaranth, quinoa, popcorn, corn tortillas, corn chips, teff, and "polenta."

• Brown rice derivatives: Mochi, brown rice syrup, rice cakes, rice crackers, riz cous, creamy rice, "Rice and Shine"™, "Creamy Rice"™, brown rice cream (a hot cereal), "Rice Dream"™ beverages (original, vanilla, almond, carob).

• Beans and legumes. All beans are allowed, including garbanzos, humus, lentils, black beans, pinto beans, etc.

• Meats: chicken, turkey, lamb, and rabbit.

• Fish: the National Academy of Sciences and the US. Food and Drug Administration (FDA) report on low- and high-risk seafood varieties. Tuna generally has low levels of environmental contaminants. Cod, pollock, haddock, Pacific halibut, flounder, ocean perch, and sole are found in deep offshore waters, so they're also low in chemical contaminants. However, ocean-caught salmon is notoriously high in parasites and should be fully cooked to destroy worms and amoebas; it is, however, otherwise free of contaminants. Canned tuna is rarely a cause of food-borne illness unless mishandled by food preparers. Beware of shrimp, though, because these scavengers of the sea are frequently mishandled in the market or in the home. As an extra precaution, consumers may want to reheat shrimp to destroy any possible bacteria or parasites. Shrimp is often treated with sulfites before they arrive on the market; this can provoke severe reactions in sulfite-sensitive patients. Within minutes of consumption, such patients will experience difficulty breathing. Such reactions have, on occasion, proven lethal, especially among asthma patients. The greatest number of illnesses from fin fish come from the tropical varieties: mahi-mahi, bluefish, barracuda, grouper, and tropical snapper.

Fresh water fish from the Great Lakes (as well as whitefish from Santa Monica Bay, Puget Sound, and Chesapeake Bay) may carry undesirable levels of chemical contaminants. Swordfish can carry elevated mercury levels and should be avoided, especially by women of child-bearing age.

The highest-risk seafoods are mollusks -- oysters, clams and mussels -- eaten raw. The intestines and viscera are the parts that we consume, and they contain all possible kinds of contamination, natural and man-made.

Raw-fish dishes such as sashimi and sushi have become widely popular but are partly responsible for an increased incidence of parasites. For a lot of people, eating quantities of sushi is like playing Russian roulette: A "bad" moment in their life, leading to a slight decrease in the strength of the immune system, can lead to an invasion of opportunistic organisms. People with an immune-suppressed condition should generally avoid eating raw fish.

• Dairy: goat's milk, goat's cheese, goat's yogurt, butter, and eggs. For those with high cholesterol, butter and eggs should be eaten only occasionally. If this is done (and sugar and the other foods on the "no" list are eliminated), LDL (bad cholesterol) levels will fall and HDL (good cholesterol) levels will rise.

• Oils: olive oil (use only organic cold-pressed, extra-virgin olive oil (so-called pure or virgin olive oils are second-rate), sunflower and safflower oils (choose the unrefined high-oleic varieties of these oils for cooking and baking), canola oil (the newest oil in the market is also the best; it contains linoleic acid, the Omega-3 fatty acid that reduces blood cholesterol levels and prevents clogging of the arteries), and avocado, sesame and flaxseed oils. With the exception of olive oil, keep all oils refrigerated.

• Nuts, seeds, nut butters and nut milks: All are allowed except peanut and pistachio products. No peanut butter! Nuts, seeds, and nut butters should be eaten in moderate amounts, since they contain high amounts of calories and fats. For instance, one handful of cashews packs about 750 calories. Keep in mind that roasted nuts are easier to digest than raw ones. (Store all nut and seed products in the freezer or refrigerator.)

• Vegetables: steam or stir-fry all vegetables; avoid eating them raw. It is all right to have lettuce with fresh tomatoes and avocados along with a salad dressing of an allowed oil with lemon juice. Sundried tomatoes are also allowed.

• Seasonings, spices, herbs, and condiments: "Quick Sip" (a tamari-style sauce by Bernard Jensen), Bragg's Liquid Aminos, garlic, onion, sea salt (sparingly), dill, thyme, tarragon, rosemary, oregano, curry, basil, parsley, paprika, cinnamon, nutmeg, carob.

• Beverages: Pau d'Arco tea, water, water with lemon juice, peppermint and spearmint teas (excellent for digestion), Uvi Ursa™ tea and parsley tea (great for urinary tract symptoms and to help strengthen the bladder). Other herbal teas (without caffeine) should be used sparingly. Watch out for either dryness or mold content, especially if they've been stored for extended periods of time.

• Breads: don't forget, most breads contain yeast and sugar; avoid breads for the first four weeks of the eating program (except for the bread recipes in this book). After that, incorporate them very gradually into your diet. Some breads you may choose: Ponce whole rye (wheat- and yeast-free), German sourbread (wheat- and yeast-free), and Rudolph's 100% rye bread with linseed (also wheat- and yeast-free). Note that many bread recipes are contained in this book.

• Sweeteners: rice syrup, maple syrup and honey, by preference in this order.

• Chocolate substitute: carob is an excellent replacement of chocolate. It almost has no fat, is high in fiber, caffeine-free (unlike chocolate), and rich in vitamins and minerals. Just remember: It is high in natural sugars; use sparingly when using as a sweetener.

• Salt: use sparingly: sea salt, kelp powder and sesame salt. It still is sodium chloride but at least they are additive free.

• Gas producing foods: apricots, bananas, Brussels sprouts, beans, celery, prunes, wheat germ, cabbage, cauliflower, broccoli and onions. Although most of these are allowed, you should limit quantities if you suffer from flatulence. Note: charcoal, taken after meals, is helpful in moderating gas production.

As you can see from this list, you shouldn't have to go hungry to eat well. The best way to make good food choices is to think about what you eat, read the labels, and keep the Seven Principles of Healthy Eating in mind. Using these principles to guide your eating patterns will enhance your immunity and bolster a sense of well-being leading to the ultimate goal -- the "Full of Life" phase.

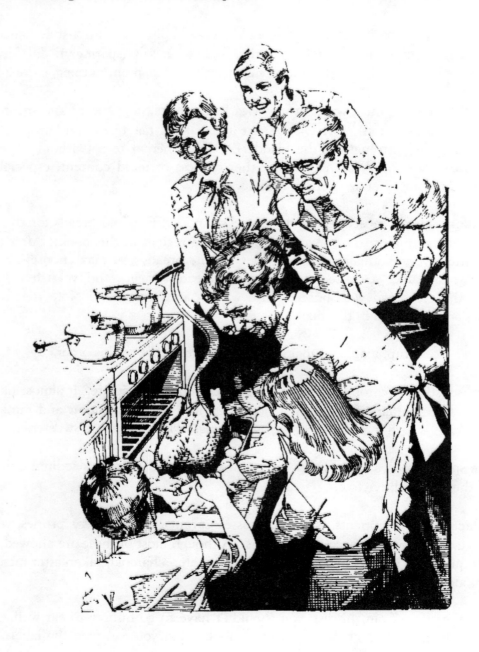

CHAPTER TWO

THE THREE DIET PHASES: MASTER KEYS TO OPEN THE GATES OF HEALTH

"He that takes Medicine and neglects to Diet himself, wastes the Skill of the Physician."
(Chinese Proverb)

PHASE 1 -- CLEANSING

Lessons of ancient medicines

One of the current problems facing modern medicine is the pressure doctors get from their patients to produce miraculous, instant results. The "magic bullet" therapy, which doctors have entertained as much as their patients, is leaving us all in the cold when it comes to introducing permanent, beneficial changes. We would each like to believe the prescription: "Take this pill first thing in the morning and feel better for the next week. Repeat as needed."

Ancient jungle medicine can teach us valuable lessons. It was the custom in so-called "primitive" tribes to put a sick person through a cleansing program: two days of fasting together with colonic-like treatments to purge the toxins. Only after this process was completed, when the absorption capacity was maximized, would a healer apply the appropriate herbs and potions. Pythagoras and Plato were among the ancient fasters who proclaimed the power and magic of a good, long fast. In fact, their prospective students were required to undertake a 40-day fast before they were allowed to study with the master. Only then did they stand a good chance of understanding clearly the complex thoughts and theories presented.

While most of us might balk at this treatment approach (lack of time and impracticality are the most frequent objections), I feel confident that almost anyone can undertake a "mini-approach" that will ensure the best possible chance of success in reaching the Full-of-Life stage.

Following this Phase 1 two-day fast, I will address the adjustment of your body to the reintroduction of food.

THE FAST: DAY 1 AND 2

Starting on the right foot

One of the most important aspects of a fast is correct preparation. You should start to prepare yourself -- both emotionally and physically -- three days before the onset of the fast by diminishing the food intake. At the same time, the regular diet should be modified to gradually lighten the load on the digestive system. For instance, it is imperative to continue eating cooked foods (stir-fried or steamed), not raw foods.

As outlined in my book, *Full of Life*, the Chinese understood the negative impact of raw foods on the spleen-pancreas, and anyone with malabsorption tendencies is likely to experience bloating, constipation, and an unpleasant feeling of fullness when eating only raw foods. So, to make it easy on the body and help the digestion as much as possible, eat cooked foods, especially prior to the onset of a fast.

The day before beginning the fast, it is very helpful to consume only soups. This will further reduce the coming fast's shock to the system.

Timing is also important. Don't begin a fast when you are premenstrual, when you are under extreme stress, or when you have a big physical event ahead. I find it much easier for myself to begin on a Saturday morning; with the weekend ahead, I can nurture my body through the different, sometimes uncomfortable changes.

At first, fasting might seem a rather unnatural thing to do. Yet, if we observe animals in nature, we learn that an early sign of acute disease is a rejection of food. Children seem to hold that wisdom too; a distressed child usually refuses nourishment that it does not need; forced feeding only aggravates conditions whose symptoms are often the result of improper feeding in the first place.

Get used to weekly fasting

(Note: *No one who has a disease should fast for more than a day without consulting their physician; further, such a person should fast only under the supervision of a doctor.)*

Fasting is a science, and it takes some getting used to. I'm sure everyone has heard stories of people who have fasted up to thirty days or more. I strongly advise anyone to never attempt more than a three-day fast, except under the supervision of a medical expert. It is much safer, and more effective in the long run, to acclimate your body to weekly 24-hour fasts. Such a one-day fast can be sufficient to activate an internal house cleaning; great benefits can be achieved by repeating these short fasts weekly. Over time, those who benefit from a regular routine of such fasts may find themselves prepared to graduate to longer periods of fasting, perhaps three to seven days.

Breaking the fast is an art

Ironically, most people have fewer problems fasting than with the return to food afterwards. Part of the difficulty is emotional. When one makes the commitment to fast, it is possible to visualize the purification that is about to take place; sudden changes during the fast create awareness of the enormous effort the body is making. However, once food begins to be reintroduced food, there can be a simultaneous sense of deprivation and craving; this accompanies certain physiological changes.

Even after a one-day fast, a great amount of the body's energy is concentrated on flushing out toxins. However, this will certainly not be sufficient to lead to an immediate, total cleansing. Most of us have poisoned ourselves for many years, so it shouldn't be surprising that many 24-hour fasts will be required to accomplish significant cleansing of the system.

It is of the utmost importance that a fast -- no matter how short it is -- be broken in a sensible way. Break the fast with vegetable juices, steamed vegetables, and brown rice. Keep it simple. Do not consume animal products (meat, fish, butter, milk, cheese, or other high-calorie, high-fat substances such as nuts and seeds) on the day after a fast. Make it easy on the digestive system. Definitely do not consume a starch-protein combination on the day after a fast.

Multitude of subjective symptoms during and immediately after the 2-day fast

For many of us contemplating a fast -- even one as short as 24 hours -- the immediate reaction is that we will probably never live to see the next day's light. We don't want to be poor and sick, but we definitely don't want to be without food, either. Ironically, most of us actually overeat most of the time, thereby directly shortening our life spans. Recent studies bear this out: Laboratory animals fed starvation diets live much longer than well-fed animals!

So, don't be afraid to start this fast. Instead, look forward to studying the various changes, objective and subjective, that your body will go through during this two-day event.

The release of toxins during fasting is well-described in Chapter 12 of *Full of Life*. A toxic headache (easily distinguishable from other types of headache) is the most common and immediate symptom of the release of toxins in the body.

A toxic headache is usually located either above the eyes (frontal) or in the top of the head (the feeling of wearing a helmet). One might also feel low on energy; depending on the extent of the clean-up that is underway in your body, one could feel either slightly fatigued or "like a bulldozer ran over you." Muscle pains, especially in the neck (we have a nice word for this: fibromyositis) and lower back, can make you think you need to visit your chiropractor. Hold off for awhile; the body is not capable of holding an adjustment at this point.

Arthritic-like pains, too, can strike with some intensity, especially in the small joints. The nose may start running, and the immediate assumption is that it's the onset of a cold. It's not! Even coughing up green mucus doesn't necessarily constitute an infection. When in doubt, let your doctor do a culture.

A most important symptom, almost always present during and after a fast is constipation. Since most of us already have problems of malabsorption and maltransportation in our digestive systems, the release of a high concentrations of toxins will initially aggravate these conditions. It is not unusual for bowel movements to stop altogether for this two-day fasting period. Bad breath is another common symptom of the release of built-up toxins.

One common but important psychological symptom of the body's intense effort at this time can be an increased tendency toward irritability and anger. In fact, such expressions arise from the difficult work of the liver, which is challenged and can be temporarily overwhelmed in its task of processing and neutralizing the sudden deluge of toxins. You might not be up to acting quite like the nicest person in the world at this point, but hang in there; you will soon have your chance!

Objective symptoms as proof of changes

Certainly it pays to listen to the body's subjective symptoms; however, the body also provides us with objective tell-tales of its internal workings, struggles, and changes. If there is one thing the doctor lost in the transition to the high-tech world of medicine, it is the capacity to look at the tongue and read from it, as from a book, the changes that are happening in the deep parts of our bodies.

Check your tongue first in the morning, before you've eaten or brushed your teeth. A healthy tongue can have a trace of thin, white fur all over its surface, but it shouldn't be cracked (although some tongues can have hereditary cracks), dry, or reddish. Some of us might already normally have a thicker white or yellow fur on our tongues. During this first two days of fasting (and even later on) the tongue will serve as a mirror of our internal cleansing program.

Figure 2 shows the different locations of the organs on the tongue. Notice that all the organs of excretion -- liver, kidneys, large and small intestines -- are associated with the lower third of the tongue. The changes created by this diet will be most dramatically obvious here. During the first two days, expect a heavy coating on this part of the tongue.

Sometimes the entire tongue reflects an mirror image of our internal changes, so keep in mind that the thicker and more yellow the coating is, the more toxins are being excreted. Even if you brush or scrape this coating off in the morning, it will return during the day, no matter how hard you try to clean that tongue. So, don't worry; make it a habit to chart the appearance of your tongue during the time-span of this cleansing phase.

The body will produce other objective symptoms during the cleansing process, including loss of head hair, skin changes, and weakening of fingernails.

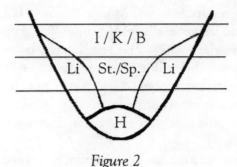

Figure 2

Location of the Organs on the Tongue
I = Intestines, K = Kidney, B= Bladder, Li = Liver, St.= Stomach, Sp. = Spleen, H= Heart

Supplements are a big help during these two days

There is considerable controversy over whether one should take vitamins or supplements during short-term fasting. In reality, all that is necessary is to use common sense. Yes, we know that positive changes we are experiencing are accompanied by discomfort, but this doesn't necessarily mean that we have to act like martyrs or heroes as we suffer in silence. Even if you understand that this process is relatively brief and self-limiting, I think that you owe it to yourself to help process along as smoothly as possible.

Dealing with headache, constipation, irritability, and pain effectively drains much of your energy and, therefore, the strength of your immune systems. Often, I have seen that patients will catch a cold or experience a flare-up of herpes simplex symptoms because of a weakened immune system and an increased susceptibility to attack. Therefore, in addition to making a short fast much more comfortable, vitamins can protect the body from effective invasion by viruses, yeasts, or bacteria. In short: you need all the help you can get!

A key vitamin you will want to take during this initial fasting period is a liver cleanser. What chlorophyll does for plants, the liver does for people. It has been called "the wheel of life" because a well-functioning liver is vital to a healthy well-functioning body.

There are foods and herbs that stimulate liver function and bile production; others reduce inflammation and act as detoxifiers. Some fruits (such as avocados, grapefruit, papaya, and cherries) have a beneficial influence on the liver. Bitter teas made from dandelion, devil's claw, or artichokes are excellent stimulants for this organ.

One of the most useful medicinal herbs for regenerating the liver is milk thistle (Sylibum marianum), also referred to St. Mary's thistle. This widespread herb is found on uncultivated ground and in waste places throughout Europe and has been naturalized in California and in the Eastern US. The seeds have been used medicinally for over 2,000 years. In ancient times, the milk thistle was said to relieve congestion in the liver, spleen, and kidneys. The active component (sylimarin) of this plant alters the outer liver membrane and inhibit toxins from entering liver cells. Besides this protective effect, milk thistle also has a curative effect, which has been demonstrated in studies of alcohol-induced liver damage. (Ref. 1)

Red beets and black radishes are also known to rejuvenate the liver. Individuals taking medication on a regular basis should consider a "beet cleanse" once a week. Beets are very high in fiber and stimulate digestion without causing cramping. The red food color of beets cannot be digested by humans, so expect stools and urine to be red. (Use this bit of information as a tool to time the speed and effectiveness of your digestive tract!)

Agrimony or sticklewort and peppermint are widely available herbs that improve the flow of the bile. Peppermint's active ingredient is menthol, which is eliminated via the liver and gallbladder. Menthol activates the secretions of these organs and stimulates

Ref. 1: Hikino and Kiso. 1988. "Natural products for Liver Disease" pp. 39-27. In "H. Wagner, H. Hikino and N.R. Farnsworth. Economic and Medicinal Plant Research. Vol. 2, Academic Press, New York.

bile secretion nine-fold. Peppermint is clearly indicated for anyone who's had a gall-bladder removed; however, anyone suffering from malabsorption (and who doesn't?) will benefit from this wonderful herb.

Herbal laxatives do have their place

It is obvious from these symptoms that you should do anything possible to help your liver eliminate toxins. The liver is the factory that processes the poison; the intestines, kidneys, and bladder are the pipelines that evacuate the debris to the outside world. Knowing how the system works leads us to the understanding that we must help facilitate our bodies' work on both levels.

For instance, while some health professionals might tell their patients not to worry about constipation in those first two days ("Every-thing will be all right," they say, "once your body has adjusted."), I cannot see much merit in keeping the toxins (or, if you prefer, poison) in the body any longer than absolutely necessary. Poisoning oneself deliberately is foolish.

I customarily advise my patients to take a natural herbal laxative during this beginning stage. My favorite is AloeV Root ™, from the aloe plant not aloe juice. Taking one tablet at the end of dinner is sufficient to enable most people to enjoy a good bowel movement; for others even this too much and can cause loose stools. So, use Aloe V in a flexible way. One day you might need one tablet; sometimes, rarely, you might need another after breakfast.

I do not recommend psyllium husk or metamucil as laxatives. Although they are highly effective at pulling toxins out of the body, they require a lot of water to do this. If one is constipated, it indicates a lack of water in the digestive tract, and psyllium husk can ultimately create further blockage and cause bloating and abdominal pain. Rather use psyllium for diarrhea. For constipation, it is preferable simply to increase the amount of fiber in the diet by eating more fibrous foods. (See Table 1 for a list of high-fiber foods.)

Another approach to dealing with constipation is to use a "stimulant purgative" such as cascara, senna and rhubarb, or buckthorne . Stimulant purgatives should not be used by persons with colitis. High doses of Vitamin C (up to 10,000 mg ester-C, buffered powder and more) are also very effective and a personal favorite. The mildest of the laxatives, licorice root, can be used for children. It can be taken in tea or in capsules, and can be used during pregnancy.

Poor diet and emotional problems are common causes of constipation; these need to be corrected prior to using these natural laxatives with children. Homeopathic laxatives are excellent for anyone: Hydrastis 6C, Nux Vomica 6C, and Bryonia 6C are my favorites, prescribed according to homeopathic principles (See my book, *Human Condition: Critical*).

After digesting the above information, you are now ready to start walking on the diet road to health!

Table 1
TOP SOURCES OF HIGH-FIBER FOODS

- Bran cereals, green peas
- Lima beans, kidney beans, chick peas
- Strawberries, raspberries, blackberries, cherries
- Broccoli, Brussels sprout, spinach, carrots
- Corn on the cob, corn kernels
- Almond nuts, walnuts, Brazil nuts

DAY 1: DISTILLED WATER EXCLUSIVELY!

If you were to refer to distilled water as "dead" water, devoid of minerals, you would be making a classic mistake. Waters other than distilled, called "hard water," contain inert, inorganic minerals that can overburden your kidneys and lead to atherosclerosis. On this first day of fasting, consuming pure distilled water will enable you to flush out a considerable amount of toxins, putting you squarely on the right path. Drink as much as you can; take a large bottle to work. Add some lemon to your water: it makes it more palatable and helps flushing the toxins out. Don't think that you will not be able to go to work. You will be pleasantly surprised at the amount of energy you will experience.

As a rule, most people drink far too little and eat far too much; no wonder toxins are impacted in most of our bodies. This is an opportunity to turn the tables -- to the benefit of your body and its dehydrated cells!

DAY 2: VEGETABLE JUICES!

Freshly-squeezed vegetable juices -- but not fruit juices -- will lead you on to the further wonders of cleansing. As with water consumption on Day 1, drink copious amounts. Carrot and red beet juice have a wonderful liver-cleansing effect and should be high on your list. But allow yourself some variations: you can make prepare most any combination: carrots, garlic, ginger, celery, beets, green leafy vegetables, etc.

Other fast foods of the future are the green juices: barley and wheat grass juices. Crushed when they're about five inches high, both of these are rich in chlorophyll, minerals, protein, and vitamins. Since not everyone has a health food store in their neighborhood to provide these freshly squeezed juices, an excellent alternative is to use "green barley essence powder." Simply dissolve a teaspoonful of the powder in a glass of water. You can definitely use the juice thus prepared on the second day, or anytime you want later. High amounts of protein (45%) and enzymes, make these juices a primary ally in maintaining health and energy while alleviating gastrointestinal problems.

DAY 3-7

Readjusting after the fast

It is important to break a fast in a sensible way. The recipes for the first week reflect this. It is essential to stick to these guidelines to avoid a crashing down. You have been very gentle to your system, and as you emerge from this two-day hibernation, your digestion does not want to wake up with a bang. In truth, it is often easier to go on a fast then to break one. During these five days you will be iniating this diet on the heels of the two-day fast. Remember. Even as the new diet continues, cleansing symptoms emerge which make you feel worse before you will feel better. Read further.

More subjective symptoms

At this point, in the first week of your diet, you might experience a variety of symptoms.   Misunderstood, they could lead to all kinds of faulty diagnoses and mistreatments. After the acute withdrawal symptoms of the first two days, the headaches will subside, only to make room for other uncomfortable feelings. For instance, a sensation of "pins and needles" (often only on one side of the body), especially in the limbs, mimics conditions with neurological involvement and could trigger suspicions of multiple sclerosis. Instead it must be realized that these are normal signs of releasing built-up toxins following two days of fasting.

This accumulated debris can also lead to joint pains or arthralgias in almost every joint, especially in the small joints of the hands and feet. These symptoms can be mistaken for an acute rheumatoid attack, though laboratory tests will prove negative and regular anti-inflammatory medications are contra-indicated.

.ve also a tendency to move into the muscles, especially in the neck and
npting a diagnosis of fibromyositis or fibromyalgia. In fact, this is not a
, since the symptoms are merely a consequence of the toxins released from
the

By this time (day 3-7) you might crave more foods, especially carbohydrates, sugar, and chocolate. These urges are even more outspoken if you are premenstrual. However, the sluggishness also begins to disappear. The biggest danger during this period is constipation.

Since toxins will use any exit in your body, you can experience urinary, vaginal, and anal burning. It is important to not make the mistake of taking these signals for infectious symptoms; this could lead to tremendously aggravating consequences. Let your body do the flushing out and try not to interfere in this natural process of elimination.

During this first week you might already experience improved digestion with less bloating and gas, improved sleeping patterns, and bursts of energy. These positive symptoms provide a first glimpse of what the future will bring.

New objective symptoms

At any time throughout this first week, other symptoms are likely to emerge. Twitching of the big muscle groups in the thighs or arms, for instance, or annoying twitching of the eye lids, and muscular "knots" that are painful to touch or massage. These are all signs of an overworked liver, an organ unable to cope with the surplus of toxins. This can also be reflected by a dullness in the eyes: the brightness and life seems to disappear for a time. In fact, the eyes are mirrors of our internal cleanliness. As your liver start coping better with the elimination, the brightness of your eyes comes back.

The skin is also an organ of elimination, and skin changes (especially on the face), often develop during this process of toxic cleansing. (Fig. 3 shows the areas most often affected.) The areas affected will correspond to the organs most actively involved in the cleansing process, such as the kidneys, bladder, and spleen-pancreas. These skin symptoms can range from dry, red patches to hard, painful boils.

Be cautious, however, in seeking symptomatic relief. Using cortisone creams, for instance, would be a big mistake, since such preparations tend to push toxins back into the body. This suppression is the worst sin of Western medicine as it goes **against the natural course of healing: from the inside of the body to the outside.** (See also my book: "*Human Condition: Critical*)

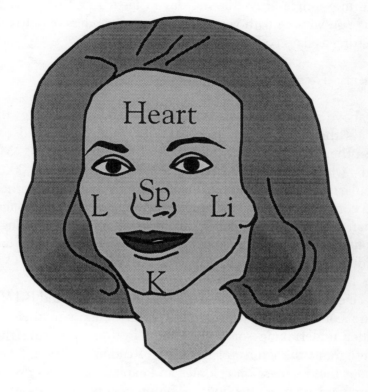

Figure 3

Location of the Organs on the Face
L = Lung, K = Kidney, Li = Liver, Sp = Spleen

Other toxin build-up symptoms found in the nails (breaking, not growing, or very thin nails) and hair (loss of head hair, dandruff which is yeast, dull and brittle hair) express the stress the body is going through. All this is reversible upon assisting your bodily excretions.

The tongue, meanwhile, will reflect further stages of detoxification. As the days go by and the digestion improves, the fur in the middle of the tongue will become thinner, less yellow, and soon disappears all together. The lower third of the tongue will also show quite a bit of activity: The fur may become thicker and more yellow, and hypertrophied, protruding taste buds may be clearly visible.

One interesting home test that can be done to evaluate the benefits of your efforts is to collect a urine sample after the first day of fasting and set it aside for a couple of weeks to settle. You will see with your own eyes the wonders of detoxification as you see the sediment setting as days go by.

Supplements: No suffering is necessary

As the above symptoms suggest, you should continue taking the supplements of the first two days throughout this first week. But you don't need to suffer needlessly because of the other discomforts related to the release of toxins. Muscular pains are easily relieved with magnesium, either in oral form (2,000 mg daily) or I.M.(Intramuscular) (1 cc twice a week) or IV. (Intravenously) together with vitamin C, Calcium, and B complex vitamins. Homeopathic remedies such as Magnesium 30C, Ruta 30C and Valerian 30C are very helpful during the day and won't produce drowsiness.

The on-and-off energy of this first week of fasting and dieting can be alleviated at this point by your doctor. S/he can give you intravenous vitamin C (15 cc vitamin C combined with 1 cc calcium, 1 cc magnesium, 1 cc B-12, B-1, B-2 and B-6), or I.M. Liver extract 1 cc combined with Folic Acid 1 cc, AMP 1 cc. and B 12, 1 cc.

If we are committed to assisting our bodies eliminate their toxins, we should seriously consider undertaking some colonic hydrotherapy during this first week and periodically throughout the course of this diet. Reading Chapter Twelve in *Full of Life* may help put your mind at ease on colonics and explain my views on their necessary role in a wellness program such as this one. The procedure takes about 45 minutes and is able to dislodge and carry toxins which have been lodged over the entire length of the large intestine. An enema, on the other hand, reaches only the lower part of the colon. The therapeutic goals of colonic hydrotherapy are to rebalance the body's chemistry, eliminate old impacted stool and bring a high concentration of anti fungal substances and friendly bacteria to every area in the colon. How do you choose a reputable colonic hygienist? Write or phone:

The American Colon Therapy Association
President Connie Allred
11739 Washington Blvd.
Los Angeles, CA 90066
Tel. (213)390-5424

Table 2 lists the supplements appropriate to this phase of the diet.

Table 2: Supplements of the Cleansing Phase

- Magnesium 2,000 mgs twice a day
- Vitamin C I.V.
- Ruta 30C
- Aloe V Tablet, one after dinner if needed
- Valerian 30C, 3 pellets at night
- Buffered powder ester-C, 10,000 mgs (3 tsp.)
- Chamomilla 30C for the withdrawal effects of coffee/drugs, 3 pellets, twice a day

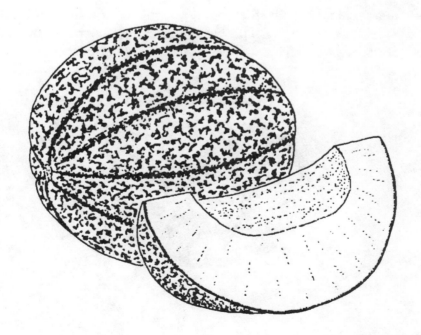

Menus Day 3-7

DAY 3 & 4: *Ted's Bean and Rice Soup*

Buy a package of "15 Bean Soup", available in all stores. Throw out the seasoning as it contains MSG, artificial flavors and artificial smoke. wash and soak the beans overnight in a large pot. The next morning, fill the pot with fresh water till 3" from the top. Boil the beans for 30' and then simmer for 4 hours. At this point, add:

- 2 cups of brown rice
- 10 cloves of garlic, chopped or minced
- 2 large onions, chopped
- 5 tomatoes chopped and/or one can of Trader Joe's marinara sauce
- 2 stalks of celery chopped
- 4 carrots chopped
- other veggies chopped as desired
- add to your taste: sea salt, pepper, bay leaves, chili, etc.

Bring to a boil and cook further for another 45' on low heat. This might look like a long process, but it's worth it. The beans are easily digestible and the soup is very nutritiously. Start preparing this soup during the second day of the fast.

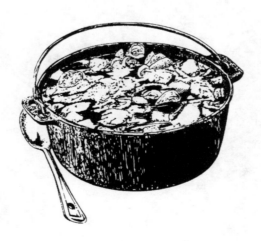

DAY 5

Breakfast

Oatmeal with Goats Milk

Prepared as usual.

※

Lunch

Beet Barley Garlic Soup

1 beet	2 cups distilled water
3 garlic clove	sea salt/pepper to taste
1 cup barley	

Place beet and garlic in blender and add to remaining ingredients.
    Serves 2-3.

Dinner

Salmon/Rice Loaf

1 cup cooked rice	1/8 teaspoon pepper
3/4 cup oatmeal	1/8 teaspoon sea salt
2 eggs, beaten	1/2 teaspoon celery salt
4 cups flaked canned salmon	1 tablespoon onion, red

Combine ingredients and place in buttered ring mold. Bake in moderate oven (350 degrees F) 30 to 40 minutes. Remove from oven and brush with melted butter. Turn onto serving platter, fill center with buttered peas and carrots.
    Serves 4.

※

DAY 6

Breakfast

Sweet Potato Pancakes

4 eggs, separated	1 tablespoon rice flour
1/4 teaspoon baking powder	1 teaspoon salt
2 cups grated uncooked potatoes	

Grate potatoes. Add egg yolks, baking powder, salt and flour and beat well. Fold in stiffly beaten egg whites. Drop from a tablespoon onto a hot well greased butter skillet. Brown on both sides.   Serve with rice syrup.

   Serves 4.

✳

Lunch

Asparagus-Cheese Tomato Sandwich

4 cooked asparagus tips	2 slices ponce bread
cayenne	softened butter
1/4 cup goats cheddar cheese/grated	

Spread slice of bread with soft butter, cover with cheese, sprinkle with cayenne, broil slowly until cheese has softened. Place tomato slice under asparagus on other slice toasted and band.

   Serves 1.

✳

Dinner

Supreme Chicken Breast

3 tablespoons curry powder	1/2 cup rice syrup
1 tablespoon black pepper	1/2 cup virgin olive oil
Juice from 4 limes	4-6 chicken breasts

Toast the curry powder in a dry sauté pan for about 1 1/2 minutes. Combine all ingredients except the chicken. Place the chicken in the marinade, cover and refrigerate overnight. The chicken breasts can be grilled, broiled or roasted.

   Serves 4-6.

✳

DAY 7

Breakfast

French Omelet with Parsley

6 eggs, separated	3/4 teaspoon sea salt
3 tablespoons minced parsley	dash pepper
2 tablespoons butter	

Beat eggs just enough to mix whites and yolks, add salt/pepper. Heat butter in an omelet pan, pour a little of it into the beaten eggs and reheat the reminder. Turn eggs into pan and as mixture cooks on the bottom and sides, prick it with a fork so that the egg on top will penetrate the cooked surface and run under the sides. While the eggs are still soft, before thickened, scatter parsley over the center of the omelet while it is cooking. Once thickened, fold over let stand a few minutes to brown and turn onto a hot dish.

Serves 6.

✳

Lunch

Squash in Casserole

3 cups mashed squash	1/2 cup butter
3/4 cups dry bread crumbs	1 teaspoon sea salt
1 1/2 cups goats cheese sauce	1/4 teaspoon pepper

Combine squash, seasonings and white sauce and stir well. Place alternate layers of squash and dots of butter in greased casserole. Top with crumbs, dot with butter and bake in moderate oven (350 degrees F).

Serves 6 to 8.

✳

Dinner

Fish Delight

1 Lb any firm lean fish	1/3 cup uncooked rice
4 large potatoes	2 green peppers, diced
6 cups hot water	2 garlic gloves, minced
2 tablespoons parsley, minced	sea salt/pepper

Cut fish into chunks, slice potatoes and onions 1/2 inch thick. Place in a kettle, add water and bring to a boil. Add rice, green peppers, parsley and garlic. Simmer about 30 minutes or until tender.

WEEKS 2, 3, AND 4 OF THE CLEANSING

Life becomes easier -- a forever-changing picture

No doubt about it, the first week was the toughest. But by the second week, there should be a lifting of the "brain fog" and its uncoordinated, cloudy thinking and lack of short-term memory. Muscles start functioning better and charley horses become rarer. There are periods of clear thinking and high energy, but it's still a roller-coaster ride: you get frustrated because you felt good in the morning but now, by three or four in the afternoon, you seem to need your second wind, but it's not coming. There's a tendency to fall asleep, too, and a nap might be necessary. But somehow you seem to recuperate by 7-8:00 p.m.

Meanwhile, sleep has become more regular, and falling asleep is much easier. You seem to be able to sleep through for hours without waking up. Though at times you may still sleep too long, more frequently you require only about six hours of uninterrupted sleep. The skin lesions start to disappear, and the hard zits on the chin fade away, sometimes leaving little scars. The skin becomes dryer as it is more able to cope with the moderating rate of toxin elimination. You seem to be less irritable, angry, and frustrated; people around you comment on how you have changed. Loss of weight is apparent. After losing first inches, most notable from around your waist, you are now losing weight at a rate that can easily be from two to five pounds a week. Vaginal or anal burning has moderated to an off-and-on pattern after the initial increase. Your cravings at this point have decreased considerably -- unless you're premenstrual, a condition which leads to a temporary aggravation of almost any symptom. Once you start bleeding, however, this aggravation miraculously ceases, and you have a clear sense of moving forward again.

As the weeks go by, bowel movements become more voluminous, easier, and more frequent. Muscle and joint pain seems to be present only when stimulated by new triggering factors: more stress, the wrong food intake because of cravings, overcast weather, premenstrual period, intake of progesterone, viral or bacterial infections, antibiotic intake, environmental sensitivities, etc. Headaches are fading toward non-existence; those that come are mild and of shorter duration.

In this new atmosphere, environmental allergies and food sensitivities will become more pronounced. As the body is purged and cleaned, it actually becomes more sensitive. It now has the clarity and wisdom to protest when something harmful is put into it; encounters with perfumes, gas, or gasoline fumes trigger off immediate headaches. Your body is coming alive, and it starts giving you clear, early warnings: "Keep me away from this food, it's dangerous! Get me out of this environment, it's killing us!"

A few weeks ago you could drink two glasses of wine and not feel any effects from it. Now a half glass seems to make you feel "spacy" and drunk; your tolerance level for alcoholic drinks, especially fermented ones (wine, champagne and beer) is way down, almost zero.

During the second, third, and fourth weeks of the program, I recommend that you continue to take the same supplements as you did during the first week. If cravings are still a problem, you should use the products described in Chapter One, page 28.

RECIPES -- DAY 8 TO DAY 28

DAY 8

Breakfast

Egg Waffles

4 eggs, separated	1/4 cup rice flour
6 tablespoons hot water	1/8 teaspoon pepper
1/2 teaspoon sea salt	2 tablespoons melted butter
2 tablespoons chopped parsley	

Beat egg yolks until lemon colored. Combine rice flour, hot water, salt, pepper and butter. Beat until smooth, add to egg yolks. Fold in stiffly beaten egg whites and parsley. Bake for 2 minutes on hot waffle iron.
Serves 2 to 4.

✳

Lunch

Cheese Soufflé Sandwiches

8 slices bread	1/2 teaspoon salt
4 eggs, separated	dash pepper
1 cup grated sharp goats cheese	dash paprika

Remove crusts and toast bread on 1 side. Combine salt, pepper, paprika and egg yolks and beat until light. Fold yolks and cheese into stiffly beaten egg whites. Heap unto untoasted side of bread and bake in moderate oven (350 degrees F) about 15 minutes or until puffy and brown.
Serves 8.

Dinner

Chicken Curry

4 Lb stewing chicken
5 cups boiling water
1 onion, cut fine
3 garlic cloves, cut fine
4 tablespoons corn oil

2 tablespoons curry powder
2 cups chicken stock
1 tablespoon rice flour
1 egg yolk, beaten

Clean chicken and cut into serving portions; cover with water and simmer until tender, 1 1/2 to 3 hours, then remove from liquid. Cook onion in 3 tablespoons corn oil, remove and brown chicken in remaining oil. Add curry powder and chicken stock, simmer for a few minutes. Combine remaining 1 tablespoon oil with rice flour and egg yolk, pour into chicken mixture gradually, stirring constantly and cook until thickened. Serve on platter surrounded with hot boiled brown rice.
    Serves 6.

DAY 9

Breakfast

Scrambled Eggs with Asparagus

6 eggs
1/2 cup cooked asparagus tips

salt and pepper
1 tablespoon butter

Add unbeaten eggs to asparagus and mix together. Season with salt and pepper. Melt butter in frying pan, add eggs and cook slowly, stirring constantly, until eggs are set. Serve on hot buttered toast.
    Serves 6.

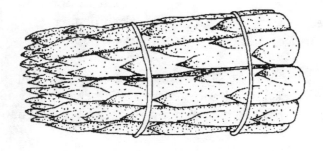

Lunch

Cream of Beet Soup

1 medium onion, minced	1 1/2 cups of water
2 garlic gloves, minced	sea salt/pepper
1 cup beets, grated	1 cup goats milk

Boil water and place onions, garlic cloves, beets and salt/pepper. Simmer until tender and add milk, heat to boiling and serve at once.
 Serves 4.

✳

Dinner

Sautéed Scallops

1 Lb scallops	1/2 teaspoon salt
1 small onion, minced	1/2 teaspoon pepper
2 garlic cloves, minced	2 tablespoons virgin oil

Wash scallops quickly and cook 5 minutes in small amount of boiling water. Drain and dry. Cook onion and garlic in virgin oil until tender. Add scallops and cook until brown. Season and sprinkle with parsley.
 Serves 4.

DAY 10

Breakfast

Oatmeal with Goats Milk

Prepare as usual.

✳

Lunch

Okra and Tomatoes

2 cups cooked okra	1 tablespoon butter
2 cups fresh tomatoes, peeled	sea salt/pepper

Simmer okra and tomatoes together about 5 minutes. Add butter and seasoning.
 Serves 6 to 8.

Dinner

Nut Vegetable Loaf

1 cup cooked tomatoes, peeled	1 cup soft bread crumbs
1 cup cooked peas	1/2 cup goats milk
1 cup diced cooked carrots	2 eggs, beaten
3 tablespoons minced onion	1 tablespoon butter
2 garlic cloves, minced	salt/pepper
1 cup chopped meat nuts	virgin oil

Combine all ingredients and turn into virgin oiled loaf pan. Bake (350 degrees F) for 1 hour.

Serves 8.

DAY 11

Breakfast

Bean Sprout Omelet

6 eggs	2 tablespoons butter
1 garlic clove, minced	3/4 teaspoons salt
1 cup bean sprout	1/8 teaspoon pepper

Beat eggs just enough to mix whites and yolks; add salt and pepper. Heat butter in an omelet pan, pour a little of it into the beaten eggs and reheat the remainder. Turn eggs into pan and as mixture cooks on the bottom and sides, prick it with a fork so that the egg on top will penetrate the cooked surface and run under the sides. While the eggs are still soft, but thickened, sprinkle bean sprouts and fold over, let stand a few minutes to brown and turn onto a hot dish.

Serves 6.

✳

Lunch

Zucchini and Tomatoes Au Gratin

2 cups zucchini	1/2 teaspoon salt
3 tablespoons chopped onion	1/8 teaspoon pepper
1 large garlic clove, minced	3 cups tomatoes, peeled
3 tablespoons virgin oil	3/4 cup grated goats cheese

Wash zucchini and cut into 1/4 inch pieces. Cook onion, garlic in virgin oil, add zucchini and cook slowly 5 minutes, stirring frequently. Add tomatoes, salt/pepper. Cover and cook 5 minutes longer. Turn into virgin oil greased baking dish, sprinkle goats cheese over top and bake in moderate oven (375 degrees F) about 20 minutes.

   Serves 6 to 8.

Dinner

Chicken Paradiso

1 1/2 cups diced cooked chicken	1/2 cup chopped celery
1 cup cooked rice	1 teaspoon sea salt
1 large onion, chopped	1/8 teaspoon pepper
1 1/2 cups cooked tomatoes	buttered crumbs
1/2 green pepper, chopped	

Combine chicken, rice and tomatoes and cook for 10 minutes. Add onion, green pepper, celery and seasonings. Turn into baking dish and cover with buttered crumbs. Bake (350 degrees F) oven. 1 hour. Serve very hot.

   Serves 4.

DAY 12

Breakfast

Pecan Waffles

2 cups rice flour, sifted	2 cups goats milk
3 teaspoons baking powder	2 eggs, separated
1/2 teaspoon salt	1/2 cup chopped pecans
1/2 cup softened butter	2 teaspoons rice syrup

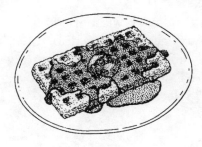

Mix and sift dry ingredients. Add milk to beaten egg yolks and butter. Add milk mixture to dry ingredients. Beat until smooth. Fold in beaten egg whites and chopped pecans. Pour about 4 tablespoons, batter into preheated waffle iron and bake 3 minutes or until steam has ceased coming from the iron. Serve hot with butter and rice syrup.

Serves 6.

✳

Lunch

Celery Chowder

4 cups cooked diced celery	1 tablespoon rice flour
1 cup cooked diced carrots	2 teaspoons sea salt
1 garlic clove, minced	1/4 teaspoon pepper
1 small onion, minced	3 cups goats milk, scaled
2 tablespoons butter	2 egg yolks, well beaten

Rub celery through a sieve. Sauté onion, garlic and carrots in butter until delicately browned and combine with celery. Blend in rice flour, salt and pepper, add goats milk gradually, stirring constantly, heat to boiling and cook 3 minutes. Before serving add egg yolks and cook 2 minutes.

Serves 6.

✳

Dinner

Fish Fillets Florentine

3 Lbs spinach	1 1/2 cups goats milk
1/4 butter	1/2 cup grated cheese
1/2 teaspoon salt	2 garlic cloves, minced
1/8 teaspoon pepper	2 Lbs fish fillets

Wash spinach in several waters and cook without adding water. When spinach is barely tender, drain and chop coarsely. Place in baking dish. Melt butter and blend in rice flour and seasonings. Add milk and cook until thickened, stirring constantly. Add cheese and continue heating until cheese has melted. Pour sauce over spinach, place fillets on top and bake in moderate oven (375 degrees F) 30 minutes.

Serves 6 to 8.

DAY 13

Breakfast

New England Griddle Cakes

1 1/2 cups sifted rice flour	1 teaspoon molasses
1/2 teaspoon baking soda	1 egg
1 1/2 cups goats milk	3 tablespoons virgin oil
1/2 teaspoon sea salt	

Sift dry ingredients together. Beat egg, sour milk and virgin oil together. Add liquid mixture gradually to dry mixture, stirring constantly to keep it smooth. Drop the batter by spoonfuls onto a hot greased griddle. Cook slowly until top is full of tiny bubbles and the underside is brown. Turn and brown other side. Serve hot with maple syrup.

Makes 2 dozen small cakes.

❊

Lunch

Broccoli Soufflé with Goats Cheese Sauce

1 cup chopped cooked broccoli
1/2 cup hot thick white sauce
2 tablespoons grated parmesan cheese
3 eggs, separated

Beat egg yolks and add to white sauce. Add broccoli and cheese. Fold in stiffly beaten egg whites. Pour into buttered baking dish and bake in moderate oven (350 degrees F) about 50 minutes. Serve with Goats Cheese Sauce (listed below).

Serves 4.

Goats Cheese Sauce

2 tablespoons butter, melted	1 cup goats milk
1 tablespoon rice flour	dash salt/pepper
3/4 cup cheddar goats cheese/grated	

Blend butter and rice flour together, add goats milk
and boil until thickened. Add seasonings and cheese
and continue to heat, stirring constantly until cheese is melted.

Makes 1 3/4 cups.

Dinner

Broiled Lamb Chops

8 lamb chops (1 1/2 inches thick)
sea salt/pepper

Broil chops for 9 minutes in a preheated broiler, 4 inches from heat. Season, turn and broil on the other side for 9 minutes. Season.
   Serves 4.

DAY 14

Breakfast

Herb Nut Omelet

2 tablespoons butter	8 eggs
4 green onions, finely chopped	1/2 teaspoon baking soda
1 or 2 lettuce leaves, chopped	1/8 teaspoon cinnamon
2 tablespoons dill weed	salt/pepper
1/2 cup chopped fresh parsley	2 tablespoons dill weed
3 tablespoons chopped walnuts	3 tablespoons raisins
1/2 teaspoon saffron powder	1/4 cup chopped cilantro

Preheat oven to 350 degrees. Melt 2 tablespoons butter in a large skillet with an oven proof handle. Add green onions, lettuce, dill weed, parsley and cilantro. Sauté until onion is tender. Add 2 tablespoons butter. Heat until melted. In a medium bowl, combine eggs, baking soda, saffron, cinnamon, salt and pepper. Stir in walnuts and raisins. Add to herb mixture in skillet. DO NOT STIR. Cook over medium heat until set around edges. Place in oven. Bake 20 to 30 minutes or until golden and set. Cut into wedges and serve immediately.
   Makes 6 to 8 servings.

Lunch

Cream of Corn Soup

5 cups fresh corn	2 tablespoons rice flour
2 tablespoons melted butter	2 egg yolks
5 cups goats milk	salt/pepper

Cook corn in double boiler with 4 cups of milk for 20 minutes. Blend rice flour and butter, add corn and milk mixture and salt/pepper. Cook for 5 minutes. Rub through a coarse sieve. Beat egg yolks and add the remaining cup of cold milk. Stir into the soup and cook for 1 or 2 minutes, stirring constantly. Beat and serve at once.

Serves 6.

✳

Dinner

Salmon Rolls

1 green pepper, chopped	1 1/2 cups flaked salmon
1 small onion, chopped	1/2 teaspoon sea salt
1 recipe baking powder biscuits (see section under "Breads")	

Roll biscuit dough to 1/4 inch thickness on floured board. Combine salmon, onion, green pepper and salt; moisten slightly with salmon liquid; mix well and spread mixture on dough. Roll as for jelly roll and slice 1 1/2 inches thick. Bake in greased pan in hot oven (400 degrees F) for 1/2 hour.

Serves 6.

DAY 15

Breakfast

Oatmeal with Goats Milk

Prepare as usual.

✳

Lunch

Cauliflower Soup

1 medium cauliflower	1 egg yolk, slightly beaten
4 cups boiling water	4 tablespoons rice flour
4 tablespoons butter	2 slices onion
2 cups goats milk, scaled	1 garlic clove
2 TBS goats cheese grated	dash cayenne

Cook cauliflower in boiling water, uncovered until tender. Strain, rubbing cauliflower through the sieve into liquid and add goats milk. Melt butter, add onion, garlic and sauté until tender, but not brown. Blend in rice flour, cayenne and salt, add goats milk mixture gradually, stirring constantly and cook 5 minutes. Pour gradually over egg yolk and mix well.

Serves 6.

✳

Dinner

Fricassee of Scallops

2 Lbs scallops	1 teaspoon minced parsley
2 tablespoons butter	1 onion sliced
1 tablespoon flour	2 garlic cloves, minced
1 cup stock from scallops	1 egg yolk
1 teaspoon fresh lemon juice	

Simmer scallops 5 to 6 minutes. Melt butter in top of double boiler, add onion, garlic and cook about 3 minutes, stir in rice flour and when well blended, add stock stirring constantly. Add parsley, salt and pepper. Beat egg yolk and pour a little of the hot sauce over it mixing well. Return to double boiler and cook for 2 minutes. Add scallops and lemon juice and heat thoroughly. Serve at once.

Serves 6.

DAY 16

Breakfast

Puffy Potato Omelet

3 eggs, separated	1/2 teaspoon minced parsley
1 cup mashed potatoes	1 teaspoon sea salt
3 tablespoons goats milk	

Add egg yolks to potatoes and beat until there are no lumps. Add minced onion, parsley, salt, pepper and goats milk. Beat egg whites until stiff and fold into potato mixture. Transfer to greased frying pan and bake in moderately slow oven (325 degrees F) until brown. Then turn and fold on hot platter. Serve at once.

Serves 4.

Lunch

Mediterranean Bean Soup

1/4 cup virgin olive oil

2 tablespoons tomato paste

3 medium onions, sliced

2 medium celery stalks, sliced

1 teaspoon dill weed

8 cups water (2 quarts)

1 Lb Great Northern Beans

2 medium carrots, diced

sea salt/pepper

2Tbs chopped fresh parsley

Heat 1/4 cup virgin olive oil in large saucepan. Add onions and sauté until tender. Stir in tomato paste. Cook 1 minute to blend flavors. Add carrots, celery, parsley and dill weed. Cook and stir until carrots are glazed, about 5 minutes. Add water, beans, salt and pepper. Bring to a boil. Reduce heat and cover. Simmer over low heat 1 hour or longer until beans are tender.

Serves 8 to 10.

Dinner

Mexican Tamale Pie

1 cup corn meal

4 cups water

1 teaspoon salt

1 green or chili pepper

dash cayenne powder

1 garlic clove

3 tablespoons virgin oil

2 1/2 cups cooked tomatoes

2 cups ground cooked
    turkey or chicken

1 medium onion

1 teaspoon sea salt

Cook corn meal, water and salt in top of double boiler for 45 minutes. Chop onion and pepper and fry in hot virgin oil. Add tomatoes, turkey, salt and cayenne or chili and cook until thickened. Line greased baking dish with virgin oil with half the mush, pour in turkey mixture, cover and remaining mush and bake in hot oven (375 degrees F) 30 minutes or until top is lightly browned.

Serves 6 to 8.

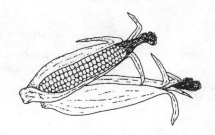

DAY 17

Breakfast

Poached Egg w/Cheese

2 cups water	dash pepper
1/2 teaspoon salt	hot buttered toast
1 egg	grated goats cheese

Heat water to simmering in a shallow pan, add salt and pepper. Break egg into a cup and slip it carefully into water. Make a whirlpool with spoon or fork. Let egg cook below boiling point for about 5 minutes or until white is firm and a film has formed over yolk. Remove egg with skimmer, drain and serve on hot buttered toast (see section "BREADS").

Lunch

Fresh Corn Soup

1 cup fresh corn	2 cups goats milk
2 cups boiling water	1 teaspoon minced onion
2 tablespoons butter	1/8 teaspoon pepper
2 tablespoons rice flour	1/2 teaspoon sea salt
finely chopped spinach	1 garlic clove, minced

Simmer corn and water together for 20 minutes. Press through a coarse sieve. Melt butter, blend in rice flour, salt, pepper, onion and garlic, add milk gradually. Heat to boil, stirring constantly, and add strained corn., Cook until thickened, about 5 minutes.
   Serves 4.

*

Dinner

Cod Creole

3 Lbs fresh cod	1 onion, chopped
2 1/2 cups cooked tomatoes	1 garlic clove, minced
6 potatoes, pared	1 teaspoon salt
3/4 cups celery & leaves	1/8 teaspoon pepper
1/4 cup virgin oil	

Cook celery, onion and garlic in virgin oil until tender, add tomatoes, salt/pepper and heat to boiling. Add cod and potatoes. Cover and summer about 30 minutes or until fish is tender basting fish frequently.

Serves 6.

DAY 18

Breakfast

Walnut Waffles

2 cups sifted rice flour	2 cups goats milk
3 teaspoons baking power	2 eggs, separated
1/2 cup softened butter	1/2 teaspoons salt
2 teaspoons rice syrup	2 eggs, separated
1/2 cup chopped walnuts	

Mix and sift dry ingredients. Add goats milk to beaten egg yolks and butter. Add goats milk mixture to rice syrup and dry ingredients. Beat until smooth. Fold in beaten egg whites and chopped walnuts. Pour about 4 tablespoons batter into preheated waffle iron and bake 3 minutes or until steam has ceased coming from the iron. Serve hot with butter and rice syrup.

✳

Lunch

Eggplant Puree Sandwiches

1 large eggplant	1 cup goats milk
1/4 cup butter	1/4 cup rice flour
1/2 cup grated Parmesan cheese	salt/pepper

Pierce eggplant in several places. Preheat oven (400 degrees F). Place pierced eggplant on oven rack and bake 1 hour or until soft. Peel softened eggplant. Place pulp in a bowl and mash. Melt butter in a medium saucepan over low heat. Stir in rice flour until smooth. Gradually add goats milk. Cook stirring constantly, until mixture is thickened and smooth, about 5 minutes. Stir in cheese, salt and pepper. Fold in mashed eggplant. Cook, stirring constantly, until thickened, about 3 minutes. Do not scorch. Serve immediately.

Makes 6 to 8 servings.

Dinner

Chicken Oregano

3 Lbs skinless chicken pieces
1/4 cup fresh lemon juice
1 tablespoon crushed
dried oregano

2 garlic cloves
1/2 cup olive oil
sea salt/pepper to taste

Place chicken pieces in a single layer in a large baking pan. Combine olive oil, lemon juice and garlic in blender. Process until mixture is smooth and creamy. Stir in oregano, salt and pepper. Pour over chicken pieces. Turn chicken to coat with marinade. Cover and marinate several hours or overnight in refrigerator. Preheat oven to 350 degrees F. Bake chicken pieces, uncovered, 1 1/2 hours or until tender. Brown tops of chicken pieces under broiler, if desired.

Serves 6 to 8.

DAY 19

Breakfast

Eggs in Onion Sauce

3 medium onions sliced
1 sweet pepper, sliced
2 tablespoons virgin oil

6 eggs
parsley
sea salt/pepper

Cook onions and sweet pepper in virgin oil until tender and brown. Beat eggs slightly, add parsley and seasoning and pour over the onions. Cook as for Scrambled Eggs.

Serves 6.

✳

Lunch

Cabbage and Celery Casserole

1/2 cup chopped celery
3 1/2 cups chopped cabbage
5 tablespoons butter
1 cup goats cheese sauce

1/4 cup dry bread crumbs
1/8 teaspoon pepper
1/2 teaspoon salt

Cook celery in 3 tablespoons butter, 10 minutes, stirring frequently.   Add cabbage and cook 10 minutes longer.   Pour into greased baking dish, add salt, pepper, and white sauce. Sprinkle bread crumbs over top, dot with remaining butter and bake in moderate oven (350 degrees F) about 20 minutes.

Serves 6 to 8.

Goats Cheese Sauce

2 tablespoons butter, melted	**1 cup goats milk**
1 tablespoon rice flour	**dash salt/pepper**
3/4 cup cheddar goats cheese/grated	

Blend butter and rice flour together, add goats milk
and boil until thickened.   Add seasonings and cheese
and continue to heat, stirring constantly until cheese is melted.

Makes 1 3/4 cups.

✳

Dinner

Tuna Supreme

2 tablespoons butter	**2 eggs, beaten**
1 tablespoon rice flour	**1 teaspoon sea salt**
1 cup goats milk	**1/8 teaspoon pepper**
1/2 cup soft bread crumbs	**2 tablespoons chopped parsley**
(see section "Breads")	
1 (7 ounce) can tuna, flaked	

Blend rice flour and goats milk until thickened, stirring constantly.   Add crumbs, tuna, parsley, seasonings and eggs.   Pour into greased shallow baking dish.   Place in shallow pan of hot water and bake in moderate oven (350 degrees F) about 40 minutes.

Serves 6.

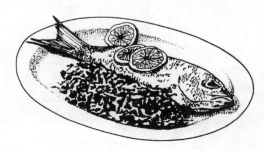

DAY 20

Breakfast

Tomato Cheese Omelet

6 eggs	2 tablespoons butter
3/4 teaspoons salt	dash pepper
2/3 cup fresh diced tomatoes	2/3 cup goats cheese

Beat eggs just enough to mix whites and yolks; add salt and pepper. Heat butter in an omelet pan, pour a little of it into the beaten eggs and reheat the remainder. Turn eggs into pan and as mixture cooks on the bottom and side prick it with a fork so that the egg on top will penetrate the cooked surface and run under the sides. While the eggs are still soft, but thickened, sprinkle diced tomatoes and goats cheese and fold over, let stand a few minutes to brown and turn onto a hot dish.

Serves 6.

✳

Lunch

Cream of Asparagus Soup

1 Lb asparagus	2 tablespoons rice flour
4 cups goats milk, scaled	1 teaspoon salt
2 tablespoons butter	1/8 teaspoon pepper

Wash asparagus, cut off tips 1 1/2 inches from top, cover with boiling water and cook uncovered until tender. Remove and set aside, add remainder of asparagus and cook until tender. Drain, rub through a sieve and add to milk. Melt butter, blend in rice flour, salt and pepper, add asparagus mixture gradually and heat to boiling, stirring constantly, cook 3 minutes. Add asparagus tips and serve hot.

Serves 4.

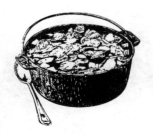

Dinner

Vegetable Loaf

1/2 cup cooked peas

1/2 cup cooked string beans

1/2 cup chopped cooked carrots

1 1/2 cups goats milk

1 cup soft bread crumbs
 (see section "Breads")

1/2 teaspoon paprika

1/8 teaspoon pepper

1/2 teaspoon sea salt

1 egg

2 garlic cloves, minced

Press peas through a sieve, cut beans into small pieces and combine all vegetables. Add milk, slightly beaten egg, crumbs and seasoning. Turn into greased baking dish and bake in moderate oven (350 degrees F) until firm.
 Serves 6.

DAY 21
Breakfast

Yogurt Scrambled Eggs

1-2 tablespoons plain yogurt

4-6 eggs

salsa (fresh)

1 teaspoon butter

dash sea salt/pepper

Beat eggs well and add seasonings. Add yogurt and stir till well blended. Melt butter in saucepan and pour in egg mixture. Cook over medium heat, stirring to fluff up the eggs as they cook. Divide the mixture into four portions and spoon a dollop of salsa over each portion.
 Serves 4.

Lunch

Winter Soup

3 tablespoons butter

1 medium onion, minced

2 tablespoons chopped parsley

celery seed

dill

2medium potatoes, diced,
  skins on

1/2 cup chopped celery

1/2 cup chopped carrots

1/2 cup peas, cooked

1 1/2 cups goats milk

2 cups stock (chicken)

sea salt/pepper

Sauté onion in butter.   Add the chopped parsley, salt and pepper and herbs.   Put the celery, carrots and potatoes into the pot and add the stock.   Simmer vegetables in the stock until tender, about 30 minutes.   Simmer uncovered.   Pour the goats milk in slowly, stirring constantly.   Heat through, but do not boil.   Add the peas and serve at once.
> *Serves 4.*

✳

Dinner

Meat Soufflés

3 eggs, separated	1 cup goats milk
2 tablespoons virgin oil	1/2 teaspoon salt/optional
1 1/2 cups minced cooked meat	1 tablespoon minced onion
(turkey or chicken)	1 garlic clove, minced

Beat egg yolks well, add virgin oil, goats milk, seasoning, meat, onion and garlic.   Beat thoroughly.   Fold in stiffly beaten egg whites.   Pour into greased custard cups, place in pan of hot water and bake in moderate oven (350 degrees F) until firm, 25 to 30 minutes.
> *Serves 6.*

DAY 22

Breakfast

Lazy Breakfast

1/2 cup cold, cooked brown rice	chopped scallion
lemon juice and soy sauce in	toasted sesame seeds
equal parts, mixed	sesame oil, optional

Put the rice in a bowl, season with the rest of the stuff to taste.

✳

Lunch

Miso Soup

3 cups prepared miso soup	3 cups cooked brown rice

Cook together 10 minutes.   Raw egg yolk may also be added.
> *Serves 4.*

Dinner

Mediterranean Sea/Fish and Rice

2 Lbs fish (halibut, cod or haddock) whole or fillet

2 cups uncooked basmati or brown rice

sesame or olive oil for sautéing

2 large onions, chopped

3 cups water

1-2 teaspoons sea salt

1 teaspoon turmeric

Marinade: **1/2 cup lemon juice**
4 tablespoons olive oil
2 cloves garlic, crushed
1 teaspoon sea salt

Combine marinade ingredients and allow fish to soak in mixture for at least 10 minutes. Sauté onions in a little oil until they are golden brown. In a large pot combine rice, onions, water, salt and turmeric. Bring to a boil, reduce to lowest possible temperature, and simmer for 45 minutes or until all water is absorbed.

Broil the fish (with all the marinade) on both sides until slightly brown. Save the extra sauce to pour over rice and fish before serving.

Cut fish into chunks and debone. Heap the rice onto a large platter with fish chunks on top and sauce poured over it.

DAY 23

Breakfast

Eggs in Bread Cups

6 slices whole-wheat bread
4 tablespoons melted butter
dash salt/pepper
1 tsp. finely minced cheese
1 teaspoon Worcestershire sauce

6 eggs
1/2 teaspoon garlic powder
1/2 cup goats grated cheddar
chives

Trim crusts from bread and press bread slices into the cups of a muffin pan. Melt butter and garlic powder in small sauce pan. Brush bread slices with garlic butter and bake in 400 degree oven for about 20 minutes, or till tasty. While bread slices bake, beat eggs and add seasonings, cheese and chives. Pour into a lightly greased skilled and cook till done, stirring frequently. Spoon cooked egg mixture into taste cups and serve immediately.

Serves 6.

✳

Lunch

Adzuke Bean Soup

1 tablespoon Eden Toasted
Sesame Oil
1 - 24 oz jar Eden Organic
Adzuki Beans
1-3 tablespoons Eden Tamari
2 cups water or stock

1 small onion, diced
1 clove garlic, minced
1 cup diced carrot
1/2 cup celery, sliced
1/3 cup parsley

Sauté onion, garlic, carrot and celery in oil for 2-3 minutes. Add adzuki, water and tamari. Cover and simmer 20-25 minutes. Add parsley. Adjust seasonings. Variation: Puree all or part before serving.

Serves 4.

✳

Dinner

Lamb Curry

2 tablespoons oil
12 oz lean lamb in 1/2" cubes
1 cup parboiled broccoli florets
1/2 cup stock
1 tablespoon cornstarch or
  arrowroot mixed with
  2 tablespoons water

1 medium onion, diced
2 teaspoons curry powder
3 tablespoons plain yogurt
1/4 lemon juice
1/2 cup peas

Heat the oil in a wok or skillet. Add the lamb and stir until the lamb and stir until the lamb is lightly browned on all sides. Add onion and curry powder and stir until well mixed.

Add broccoli, stock and lemon juice. Mix well, bring to a boil, cover and simmer 5 minutes or until lamb is tender. Stir in the peas. While stirring, slowly add the cornstarch mixture. Simmer, stirring until thick. Remove from heat. Stir in yogurt. Serve hot.

Serves 4.

DAY 24

Breakfast

Poached Eggs in a Biscuit Basket

6 large Shredded Wheat Cereal biscuits	2 cups goats milk
6 eggs	2 tablespoons butter
	dash sea salt/pepper

Gently cut the Shredded Wheat biscuits in half lengthwise. Warm biscuits in a 300 degree oven. While biscuits heat, pour goats milk into skillet and add butter and seasonings. When mixture is warm and butter melted, gently break eggs into milk mixture and cook till done, spooning some hot milk gently over the tops of the eggs to cook the top portions. Carefully spoon cooked eggs and milk over warm biscuits and serve immediately.

Serves 6.

✳

Lunch

Supreme Creamy Carrot Soup

4-5 carrots, shredded	2 cups goats milk
1 large chopped onion	2 teaspoons tomato paste
1 tablespoon vegetable oil	dash cayenne pepper
2 tablespoons rice flour	dillweed and herb salt to
2 dashes paprika	taste

Put carrots and onion in a skillet with warmed oil. Sauté just until tender. Sprinkle with rice flour and paprika and stir to combine the mixture, approximately 2 minutes over medium heat. Add goats milk and simmer for about 5 minutes, stirring continually.

Remove from heat and put carrot mixture in blender with tomato paste and seasonings. Blend on low speed until smooth.

Serves 4.

✳

Dinner

Baked Macaroni and Cheese

2 cups shredded sharp cheddar goats cheese	1 teaspoon dry mustard
2 1/2 cups goats milk	1 teaspoon sea salt
2 tablespoons rice flour	2 cups uncooked
2 tablespoons butter	buckwheat elbow macaroni

Preheat oven to 375 degrees. In medium saucepan, melt butter, stir in rice flour, mustard and salt. Gradually stir in goats milk. Cook and stir until mixture thickens slightly and mixture should coat spoon. Remove from heat. Add 1 1/2 cups shredded sharp cheddar goats cheese, stir until melted. Stir in cooked macaroni. Turn into buttered 1 1/2 quart shallow baking dish. Top with remaining cheese. Bake 20 to 25 minutes or until bubbly.

Serves 4.

DAY 25

Breakfast

Carob Chip Pancakes
(with Orange Sauce)

2 cups whole-wheat pastry flour	1 1/2 cup goats milk
4 teaspoons baking powder	1/4 cup melted butter
1 tablespoon grated orange rind	1/2 cup carob chips
	2 eggs, beaten
	dash sea salt

Mix dry ingredients together in mixing bowl. Combine eggs, milk and melted butter. Stir well. Add wet ingredients to dry ingredients, stirring till smooth. Add carob chips and orange rind and stir these ingredients through pancake batter. Cook on a lightly greased griddle.

Makes about 1 dozen 4" pancakes.

Orange Sauce for Carob Chip Pancakes

> 1 tablespoon cornstarch, more if needed
> water
> 1 - 1 1/2 cup orange juice

Dissolve the cornstarch in a little water to form a thick paste. Stir it into the orange juice in a small saucepan. Heat orange juice mixture over medium heat, stirring constantly till sauce is thickened to desired consistency. Serve hot over pancakes. *Makes about 1 -1 1/2 cups.*

✳

Lunch

Dutch Bean Soup

> 1 cup navy beans   1 small onion, grated
> 3 quarts water   sea salt/pepper
> 1 cup thick sour cream

Wash beans, cover with cold water and soak overnight. Drain and cook in water listed until they have the consistency of thick cream and have cooked down to 3 pints, add salt/pepper to taste and onion. Heat to boiling and add sour cream.
>   *Serves 7.*

✳

Dinner

Lentil Roast

> 2 cups lentils, cooked and   2 celery stalks, chopped
>   pureed   1 teaspoon sea salt
> 1 cup whole-wheat bread   1 clove garlic, minced
> 1 small onion, chopped   1 cup tomato puree
> 1 teaspoon salt

Turn out into oiled loaf pan, cover, bake 40 minutes at 350 degrees.
>   *Serves 4.*

DAY 26

Breakfast

Tapioca Omelet

3/4 cups goats milk   1/2 teaspoon sea salt
4 eggs, separated   1/8 teaspoon pepper
2 tablespoons quick-cooking   1 tablespoon butter
   tapioca

Scald milk. Add tapioca, salt and pepper. Cook 20 minutes in a double boiler, stirring occasionally. Add butter and beaten egg yolks. Fold in stiffly beaten egg whites. Pour into hot buttered skillet and bake in moderate oven (350 degrees F) 20 minutes.
   Serves 4.

✳

Lunch

Avocado Tomato Soup

1 sweet onion, small, cut   1 tablespoon lemon juice
   in pieces   pulp of 1 large avocado
1 Swiss vegetable bouillon   3 cups tomato juice
   cube

When smooth, season to taste with salt and cayenne pepper. Serve very cold. Garnish with minced chives.
   Serves 4.

✳

Dinner

Chicken Ala Tartar

1 broiling chicken   2 garlic cloves, chopped
1/2 cup virgin oil   1/2 teaspoon sea salt
4 parsley sprigs, chopped   1/8 teaspoon pepper
1 small onion, chopped   bread crumbs

Split chicken into halves and place in skillet with virgin oil. Pour over chicken, parsley, onion, garlic and salt/pepper. Simmer for 15 minutes, turning occasionally. Dip chicken into bread crumbs and broil until browned.

Serves 4.

DAY 27

Breakfast

Over the Shoulder Omelet

4 or 5 eggs	dash curry powder
1/2 cup yogurt (goats)	1/2 cup celery, thinly sliced
2 tablespoons onion, grated or green onion, finely chopped	butter
1 cup cheddar cheese (goats) grated	

Beat eggs, yogurt and curry powder till well blended. Add cheese and stir. Add vegetables, folding them thoroughly through egg mixture. Pour into buttered pan and cook over medium heat, stirring well till egg mixture is well cooked.

Serves 4.

✳

Lunch

Carrot Soufflé

3 tablespoons butter	1 cup hot goats milk
3 tablespoons rice flour	1 1/4 teaspoon sea salt
2 cups cooked carrots, mashed	2 eggs, separated
virgin oil	

Melt butter, add flour and salt. Add goats milk slowly until tickened, stirring constantly. Beat egg yolks, add white sauce slowly, then stir in carrots. Cool. Beat egg whites until stiff and fold into mixture. Pour into virgin oiled casserole or mold, place in pan of hot water and bake in moderate oven (350 degrees F) 40 to 50 minutes.

Serves 6.

Dinner

Skillet Chicken Italiano

2 teaspoons vegetable oil
1 chicken (3-4 Lbs), cut in
serving pieces

1 large onion, sliced
1 16 oz jar spaghetti sauce

Rinse the chicken pieces with cold water. Pat dry. Heat the oil in a skillet. Brown the chicken pieces a few at a time. Set aside. Pour off all oil. Return chicken to the skillet with the remaining ingredients. Cover and simmer 45 minutes or until chicken is tender. Serve with hot, cooked pasta.
Serves 4.

DAY 28

Breakfast

Oatmeal with Goats Milk

Prepare as usual.

✳

Lunch

Asparagus Casserole

3 cups cooked asparagus
4 tablespoons virgin oil
2 tablespoons rice flour
1/2 cup grated goats cheese

2 tablespoons butter
2 cups goats milk
sea salt/optional
1 garlic clove, minced

Cook asparagus just 5 minutes then place asparagus in casserole. Blend virgin oil and flour, add milk gradually and cook slowly until thickened, stirring constantly. Add cheese and salt. Pour sauce over asparagus, sprinkle with crumbs. Dot with butter and bake in slow oven (325 degrees F) 30 minutes.
Serves 6.

Dinner

Garlic Fried Fish Steaks
(with Garlic Sauce)

6 cloves garlic, crushed	1/2 teaspoon ground
4 tablespoons olive oil	coriander
2 tablespoons lemon juice	pinch of cayenne
1 teaspoon tarragon	2 Lbs fish steaks, any kind
1/2 teaspoon salt	rice flour
1/2 teaspoon pepper	virgin oil for frying

Make a paste by thoroughly mixing all the ingredients, except the fish steaks, flour and cooking oil, then rub the steaks with the paste. Refrigerate for 2 hours, then dredge the steaks in flour. Heat 1/2" deep oil in a frying pan and fry the steaks until they turn golden brown. Serve hot with Garlic Sauce.

    Serves 4.

<u>Garlic Sauce</u>

    2 heads garlic, peeled
    1/2 cup olive oil
    1/3 cup lemon juice

Place all the ingredients in a blender and blend into a thin paste.

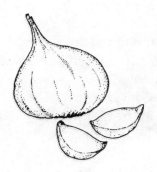

PHASE 2 -- STABILIZING

There is a feeling of renewal in the air

Congratulations! You are well on your way toward reaping the benefits of all your hard work. You can now feel your body beginning to yearn for clean food, for more protein and complex carbohydrates. Your cravings have become virtually non-existent at this point (except for an occasional premenstrual urge), and your new-found energy makes it much easier to resist these temptations.

In the event you falter (which is very human, and so a very common experience for all of us), you feel the effects of a sugar intake within five minutes. Not only does such an intake decrease your physical strength, but worse, it can dump you into an immediate depression. If you ever needed more information on how the body reacts to junk food intake, this will provide it. Your body simply does not want it any more.

You feel happier and less irritable. Your friends and family comment on your new-found vigor. Naps are not necessary anymore; instead, there is enough energy to exercise on a daily basis. Your hair is becoming stronger and shows a renewed vigor and shine with less tendency to break or fall out. Your nails are stronger; they are tough and don't break easily.

By now you are experiencing about five good days and two bad days in an average week -- quite a difference from just a short time ago when the good days were few and far between. Bowel movements are regular most of the time; you have at least one movement a day. Some may even experience one less than an hour after each meal. Mucus has cleared from the stools, and the greenish appearance has been replaced by a healthy orange color (a proof of an excellent cleansing) or by pale, less-smelly stools.

Headaches and joint pains occur only when you've made a dietary mistake. People are commenting on the brightness in your eyes. You haven't seen your chiropractor for a couple of weeks because the fibromyositis has lessened considerably at this point. You've lost a fair amount of weight -- from 6 to 30 pounds, depending on how much you needed to lose. Your skin may still be dry, but any boils have faded. Your athlete's foot is disappearing, and your acne lesions are drying up. Your tongue is clear most mornings; the only changes still happening are on the back of the tongue where a fur may occasionally be apparent in the morning. This is because you are still eliminating toxins. The condition clears of itself during the day. There is no longer any metallic taste in the mouth.

Any heart palpitations or pressures in the chest are also disappearing, since you're body has cleared out almost all of its mucus. The menstrual cycle -- absent or irregular for some time -- has suddenly become regular with normal amounts of blood loss and a minimum of pain. Your libido is coming back, your sexual energy is again a part of your reality, and any vaginal discharge is diminishing rapidly.

Dizzy spells and orthostatic hypotension have disappeared. You have more confidence driving your car, especially now that your sense of orientation is improving. Your mood swings -- once a curse to you and anyone around you -- are gone or much more manageable. You seem less irritable, more tolerant, and you hear from immediate friends that other people have commented on "what a nice person you have become."

By now, exercise has become a joy, not a chore. It is generally easier to accomplish more. Sore muscles have relaxed and adjusted, and there is a true desire in you to continue with an excellent exercise program. Your body seems to move around with more lightness and "spring." The bathroom scale agrees. Your weightloss has been considerable, so it's time to go back to those pants and dresses you stored away years ago, but never really thought you'd wear again.

If anything still hinders you, it is the "brain fag" and a seemingly increased sensitivity to certain environmental factors. At this point a lot depends on the skills of your physician. Your brainfag symptoms are an expression of a deficient toxin elimination; the sensitivities reflect a hyperactive immune system. You may still have difficulties remembering the names of friends, or you might still tend to lose the trend of conversation. Remembering what somebody told you five minutes ago or what you just read can sometimes bring you to the brink of desperation. The best strategy for continuing to decrease the brain fag and these sensitivities is avoiding the triggering factors and having acupuncture and homeopathic treatments, while continuing the supplements discussed earlier in this chapter.

Post-nasal drip can also be a bother. You're still clearing mucus from your throat in the morning, but the irritation in your throat has diminished. Coughing is rare. Sniff some salt water in the morning to clear this mucus. Often the homeopathic remedy, Kali Bich. 30C is helpful.

Watch out for warning symptoms!

The above scenario is the happy one, and one that you can achieve in normal circumstances. Alas, you are not living in a cocoon, protected from any and all noxious factors. You are a human being, living a life, and susceptible to many factors. Whether these factors will affect you negatively or not depends to a large degree on your ability to recognize danger signs and on the ongoing help that your physician is able to offer you.

So, what are the danger signs, the warning symptoms that you should look for? They are what we call in Chinese medicine the "liver and spleen-pancreas symptoms." Since, at this point, your body is so finely tuned, you will now be able to recognize these symptoms immediately. Your body is no longer numb and oblivious to its own pain and illness; it is no longer willing to suffer perpetual abuse. Instead, it provides clear signals for you and your physician to read.

The liver signs include irritability, anger, frustration, insomnia, muscle pains, breaking of the nails, graying of the hair, blurred vision, teary eyes, nausea, high stomach pains, headaches on top of the head, and menstrual irregularities.

Spleen-pancreas symptoms are loose stools alternating with constipation, water retention, loss of muscle tone, cellulite, loss of short-time memory and concentration, sugar and carbohydrate cravings, anal, urinary, or vaginal itching and burning, itching and swelling of the eyelids, thrush, worrying constantly, obsessive compulsive behavior (especially for cleanliness), butterfly rash on the cheeks, and other dry rashes on the skin.

Along with any changes on your tongue, you must be wise enough to recognize these symptoms for what they are: a temporary return to Phase 1. Do not neglect to address the indications immediately, or you will lose ground day by day.

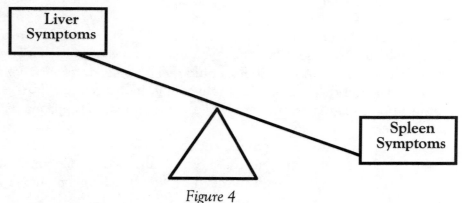

Figure 4
Warning Signs: Imbalanced Spleen and Liver Symptoms

Cut down on your supplements

It may have become obvious to you that, with the improvement you have experienced, many of the supplements you've been taking are no longer needed. Of course, if you still have Phase 1 symptoms, you should continue to take those supplements that are helpful for your particular complaints.

The next step is to focus on the brain fog and the environmental sensitivities. For an improved memory, I recommend 500 mg of choline, taken three times a day. Choline is the precursor of lecithin; it's available at your health food store. Phenylalanine is another amino acid useful in short-time memory loss. Another very useful supplement are the leaves of the Ginkgo biloba tree (the world's oldest living tree species). Several studies have shown the positive effects of the ginkgo on the impaired mental patient worldwide. Short-term memory, lack of vigilance, and depression have each been successfully ameliorated with a dose of 40mg three times daily.

Vitamin E 400 I.U. ("International Units") combined with Selenium (100 mcg) is an excellent combination for developing resistance to environmental sensitivities. Desensitization may or may not be of help to a particular patient. When one is highly reactive to the environment, it indicates that the immune system is already overactive. Often a patient reacts negatively to the desensitization shots because such therapy adds extra work to an already stressed immune system. The best desensitization method is the EPD or Enzyme Potentiated Desensitization, introduced in this country by Dr. Mc Ewen from England and practiced by physicians throughout the country. Only one injection every two months is required and usually after 3 to 4 injections the allergy shots are gone. Consulting your doctor is necessary to see if other modalities (homeopathy, acupuncture) are more helpful.

PHASE 3 -- FULL OF LIFE

> *You want to keep this feeling*

Four weeks of hard work, adjustment, feelings of being deprived, and enduring an array of objective symptoms have finally paid off. Gone are the ups and downs in energy; gone are the mood-swings and cravings. Now there is a constant feeling of being on the top of the world!

At this stage, you should feel quite comfortable in your ability to do the right things for yourself. In the past, unfortunately, when you didn't feel good, you were not inclined to exercise, to eat well, to be upbeat, or to effectively take care of yourself. Now things are different. You have even passed the point of saying to yourself, "I feel deprived because I can't eat this, but I want to continue eating this way because I feel too good!" Now it's simply: "I never want to go back to the brain fog and those feelings of sluggishness and inertia!"

After the cleansing and stabilizing phases, you are seldom tempted to return to the old foods and the old ways. When you do "cheat" on your food, you react immediately, experiencing feelings of physical and mental fatigue, a heaviness in the stomach, and a general feeling of malaise. The good news is: You can pull yourself out of such a state much faster than in the past by returning to your excellent lifestyle.

Exercise, too, comes much more easily at this point, as you enjoy your renewed strength and stamina. People comment on how well you look, how your eyes have this renewed life in them, and how balanced you have become emotionally. Your weight should be close to ideal now; in fact, people start telling you that you're too skinny! (You know you've made it when you hear that type of comments.) I am amazed that even the patients themselves start to worry when their weight drops to the level it was when they were 18 -- as if it's somehow natural to be 20 pounds overweight by the time you reach 40!

Enjoy your new body. But remember: It's not how much you weight that's important, but how well you feel, and I've seen very few people who were 30 pounds overweight and felt great.

Another benefit that comes with this new body of yours is that you don't seem to catch all those sniffles and colds like you used to. This is the clearest sign of a renewed and vigorous immune system, able to defend you even in the toughest situations. Even stress is not perceived as stress anymore, but as a challenge! You don't feel like a strip of elastic that is being stretched to the max., ready to snap at the slightest new demand. Instead, you look at situations calmly, see what you can do about them, and act. In other words, this is what life is supposed to be: a celebration!

Supplements to keep your energy

Because most of your symptoms have disappeared, many of the supplements can, too. Instead of struggling to overcome illness, fatigue, and depression, you are now more concerned with maintaining your that new-found vigor and sense of well-being. You know that the key to your health and happiness is a strong immune system. So, there will be a place in your lifestyle for ongoing supplements to ensure your continued robust condition.

Several supplements described in my book *Full of Life* are appropriate. Among the best are vitamin C (4,000 mg daily as a maintenance dose), coenzyme Q10 (60 mg daily), beta carotene (25,000 I.U daily), vitamin E (400 I.U daily), and selenium (100 mcg daily). Forget those multivitamins; most often they contain too little of anything to bring any benefits to health.

As time goes on, each of us has to keep an eye on any symptoms that might still be present. Most of the time, they're a sign of a build-up of toxins, stress, or environmental stress. Recognizing and avoiding the triggering factors of these conditions will continue to be essential.

CHAPTER THREE

LIFE ON THE ROAD

"Let food be your medicine, and let medicine be your food." -- Hippocrates

Being on cruise control is dangerous

Once you've decided what's right to eat, you will encounter a new and fearsome obstacle: How do we hold to our full-of-life diet when we're dining out? Eating out has become such a fact of life for many of us that our continued health and balance depends on being able to control what we eat in the restaurant environment.

Being a health-oriented individual with a particular set of limitations, you will find it necessary to approach the restaurant world as if you were navigating your ship through a minefield. Left to our own devices, most of us would have no worries about regulating our intake of fat and calories, about consuming plenty of fruits, avoiding sugar, and all the rest of it -- if it were not for this "other" life.

When we eat out, it is almost as if we switch on the automatic pilot or cruise control. Suddenly we seem to hear a disembodied voice hypnotically controlling our actions, telling us, "You have now entered a restaurant zone. Please relinquish all control. Relax. Please do not ask questions."

The usual response to this invisible but not-so-subtle pressure is to jettison all common sense and abandon our own proven healthy food standards. But must it really be this way? Do we really want give away all of our efforts and understandings and efforts for a quick fix that will cause us to suffer again tomorrow, and maybe for much longer than tomorrow? We know what happens when we eat incorrectly, so what's stopping us?

The question for each of us must be: am I willing to apply my healthy-eating precepts each and every time I place an order? Am I really willing to commit to this, despite the feelings that say, "Awe, the hell with it! Bring on the `goodies,' I'll deal with reactions later. Besides, I can always fast for a day or take a colonic tomorrow to clean out the toxins."

It is obvious that each of us is ultimately responsible for our own bodies. To be a good steward of the vehicle we've been given, we must take control of health, and this full-of-life diet is a way of doing this. Let's look at some proven strategies that will help us along the way.

Tips and tricks to control our eating environment

These are a few approaches that have helped me and many of my patients. Perhaps they'll work for you.

• Plan in advance. Try to find a restaurant in your area where you can order according to your desires. If you have to eat in a restaurant that is unfamiliar, ask friends about it or stop by to review the menu in advance. You'll quickly have all the information you need. Red flags on the menu are words like "fried," "crispy," "breaded," "au gratin," and "batter dipped" since these mean extra calories and fats. Rather look for "broiled," "steamed," "stir-fried," or "poached."

• Avoid the really busy places. You don't want to dine in a place where the waiter takes away your plate before you're finished with it. If your waiter is hurried, it will also be more difficult for her or him to see that your special needs are met. Instead, look for a quiet, intimate place that provides a positive atmosphere for easy digestion. The influence of such a subdued ambiance will also help you eat more slowly, allowing a comfortable length of time for proper chewing. Besides the obvious gratification for the taste buds, thorough chewing is essential in processing foods like starches, whose digestion starts in the mouth.

• Set spending limits. Bring only a limited amount of cash when you go out to eat, and avoid paying the bill with a credit card. This way you'll have less tendency to over-order, over-eat, and over-spend.

• Be first to order. That way, you'll be less influenced and tempted by what others order. Instead, you set the trend and avoid the power of suggestion. You might even steer others of your party in a more positive direction, "breaking the ice" on the healthy approach and prompting them to consider their choices from a similar angle.

• Say no to free munches. Don't allow bread or chips to be placed on the table. Ask your wait person to remove it before you begin to order. If you're dining with someone who's interested in the free munches, let the others take some, then have the wait person remove the rest before you get seduced into taking some yourself.

• Bring your own salad dressing. Since you want to avoid both vinegar and creamy dressings, bring along a small jar of dressing of your own creation. In this book, you'll find several mouth-watering dressings that are low in calories and won't cause fermentation in your digestion of other foods.

• Order appetizers. Instead of a full-course dinner, order a couple of appetizers. A shrimp cocktail and a salad can be very satisfying, as well as pleasing to the eye. Such a moderate approach is good for digestion and helps one avoid the post-pandrial fatigue that hits so many of us in the afternoon.

• Don't eat when you're hungry. Don't arrive too hungry; eat a healthy snack before you go to a restaurant. You can soften your appetite by filling up on mineral water with a little taste of lemon before the meal. After all, our idea of how much food we really need is exaggerated.

• Avoid exotic and "gourmet" sauces. Especially avoid those prepared with wine, Armagnac, cognac, butter, or cream. Instead ask for extra lemon, garlic, ginger, and other delicious condiments that will entertain your taste buds.

• Stick to the essentials. Order soup, meat or fish, and vegetables or carbohydrates. Keep it simple, and keep in mind that it's easier to control your food intake before it arrives on your plate than after. Once the different foods are smiling in your face, it becomes a Herculean task not to eat them.

• Get the check with the food. Asking the wait person for the check when the food is served reduces the likelihood of ordering dessert and may prevent you from having to hear your waiter recite his inventory of mouth-watering confections. You will also avoid a lot of calories, fats, bad food combinations, and a good dose of indigestion.

• Talk with your wait person. Good communication with your wait person is your best mine-sweeper. Try not to feel like you're pestering your waiter with your special requests. Understand that eating well and knowing what's in the food you order are reasonable expectations. State your concerns and ask your questions in a friendly but convincing matter. Waiters and chefs sometimes have little understanding of the effects certain foods or ingredients have on their customers. You are often the only one who can guide them. Your responsibility (in caring for your health) is to explain that even small amounts of particular foods can cause you big problems. For instance, if you are dining in a Chinese restaurant, you could ask them to omit MSG, soy sauce and sugar, standard ingredients in most Chinese meals. Often these components might already be in the prepared foods, so the chef might ignore your requests, regarding you as being eccentric.

Often I exaggerate. Something in the line of, "Last time I had MSG in a restaurant, they had to bring me to the emergency room." Dramatic but helpful. If a particular restaurant fails to honor your choices, find one that does. "The customer is king" is not merely a form of courtesy. Right now, it is essential to your health.

• Make your own lunch when possible. If you don't have business lunch obligations, prepare a healthy lunch the evening before. This way you have complete control over the combinations, the ingredients, and you'll save a bundle.

Table 2 recapitulates the above rules, stick to it and miracles happen!

TIPS TO CONTROL YOUR EATING ENVIRONMENT
- Plan in advance
- Avoid busy places
- Set spending limits
- Order first
- No to free munches
- Bring your own salad dressing
- Appetizers can replace a meal
- Avoid gourmet sauces
- Stick to the essentials
- Get the check with the food
- Talk with your waiter
- Make your own lunch

Table 2

Flying can be hazardous to your health

We take a surprising number of health risks any time we fly on a commercial plane flight. Besides the obvious danger of having 30,000 feet of open space beneath your seat, there's carbon dioxide, fungi, bacteria, and generally poor air quality. To top it all, the food you're served is bound to nutritionally unsound, aggravating the other rigors and stresses of flying. Airplane food is rich in fat, cholesterol, sugar, and preservatives; due to improper storage, it can often harbor bacteria. Of course, the food labeling in the air is as misleading as food labeling on the ground. On one national flight, I recall being presented with an "all natural" apricot cluster cookie. My first thought was, "Great! This airline really cares what people are consuming." Alas, it pays to check the backside of the label. As it turned out, this particular "all natural" product contained dried apricots (which alone is more than sweet enough), caramel, sugar, brown sugar, and corn fructose. In other words, five sweeteners! How, I wondered, did this cookie deserve the name "all natural."

I have had patients, who survived extended trips to third-world countries without getting sick, pick up an army of parasites on the flight back. They didn't know that the airline got its meals from the very country they had traveled to, where many of the food handlers were chronic, asymptomatic parasite carriers. How do you avoid this apparent trap?

The golden rule of air travel says, when you take an airplane, bring your food. If you can't, you can do yourself a favor by ordering meals in advance (a couple of days is usually enough). Most airlines offer a special vegetarian (mainly fruit) or seafood plate without added cost. So, being in an airplane doesn't necessarily mean giving up control of your diet and health.

"Food pushers" are deadly for good intentions

I'm sure most of us have an Aunt Daisy, who looks forward to seeing us and always seizes an opportunity to make us her favorite cookies. She insists we take some, and the look in her eye clearly doesn't want "no" for an answer. And, because you don't want to hurt the feelings of this sweet old lady and because your will power has gone to sleep, you eat eight cookies. This creates a contented glow of satisfaction in Aunt Daisy's eyes, but it turns you into a depressed wreck with a food hangover the next day.

How do you handle Aunt Daisy and the others who mean well as they urge unwanted food on you? What should you do when your spouse sits next to you watching TV and insists on having that crunchy ice cream? And what do you do when a colleague at work brings in a plate of fresh-baked cookies? How do you avoid the cookies while you avoid hurting feelings by rejecting a culinary labor of love? And the problem is compounded because the food is really tasty-looking and you really do want some!

Although they mean well, these "food pushers" threatened to kill off all our good intentions. Both communication and assertiveness are necessary to deal with this problem. To most of us, such skills don't come naturally, but we can acquire them without alienating our family or friends.

The first step is *awareness*. Offering food is often automatic; neither the person doing the offering nor the guest thinks much about the exchange, but usually, out of social grace, we accept.

As we raise our level of consciousness in this particular area, we may be surprised at how many other food temptations we're faced every day. Observe others, too, and see how often they're tempted by the well-meaning offers of food pushers. And learn about the tactics Aunt Daisy is using to put this unwanted food in your mouth. "Don't you like my food? I spent hours making it. I remember when you were small, it was your favorite. If you don't eat it, it will spoil, and I'll have to throw it out. Don't you love me anymore?" The list of guilt stimuli goes on.

This is where you need to develop a critical skill: *communication*. If your level of assertiveness is not enough to get you out of trouble, more delicate communication skills should be the next weapon in your arsenal. You've got to stand up for your rights. Just because someone insists you take this food, doesn't mean you don't have the right to refuse it. However, the way that you communicate this refusal can neutralize any uncomfortable feelings between the parties involved.

The key is to not become offended or angry because someone sets a food trap for us. Explain in a calm, pleasant tone that you have decided to pay more attention to your food intake. Try something like: "I am trying to lose some weight," or "I haven't felt very energetic lately, so although I'd love to eat these cookies, it's more important for me at the moment to take good care of myself." You'll be surprised how you can get the other person's attention and even earn a little admiration and respect.

Body language is key to effective communication. As you're offering your kind refusal, you can give Aunt Daisy a hug and dispel all of the sweet old lady's fears that you don't love her anymore. Don't show an angry, impatient face or make unnatural hand gestures. Such responses can create a very unpleasant atmosphere, making for upsets that can even lead to an increased food intake.

Another idea is to take Aunt Daisy to a natural-foods restaurant where you can be in control, and she can see that you're not alone in your preferences. Not only is it a lovely gesture to take Aunt Daisy out, but you'll avoid all those temptations that threaten to ruin all your good intentions. (If you don't feel confident that you can pull off such a performance, rehearse it in private, practicing your speech until it comes spontaneously and naturally.)

When invited over to friends for dinner, explain in advance what your dietary restrictions are. If they're really friends, they'll respect your wishes and cheerfully accommodate you. You can even offer to bring a particular dish or offer suggestions of nice, "safe" recipes.

Whether, in reality, the food pusher is Aunt Daisy, a co-worker, a friend, or your spouse, your defense tactics will be the same. A positive but assertive approach will win their respect and keep you on track. And be sure to thank your "food pushers" profusely for showing so much understanding and being such a great help. At such moment, what else can they do but give up the fight graciously?

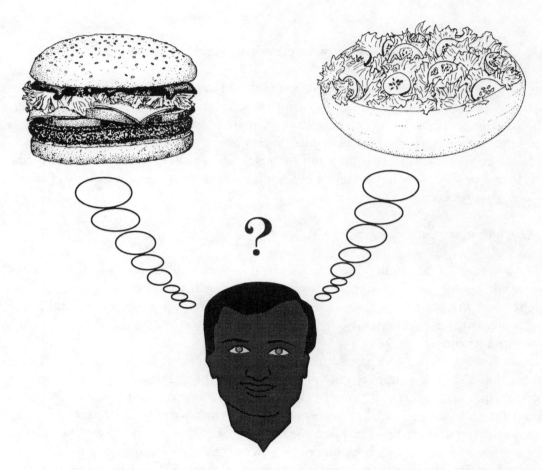

Life on the road: decisions, decisions, decisions...

CHAPTER FOUR

KEY PROFILE OF FOODS

"Do you have an appetite for a change in your life?"

Quinoa, amaranth, and couscous: how to pronounce and eat them.

Mention quinoa and amaranth in conversation and eyebrows are likely to be raised. Are these strange animals or maybe the latest in Japanese cars? Maybe they're exotic flowers from the Middle East? In fact, both should be household words in our dietary language. And the foods they signify ought to be regular guests on our tables.

Some recipes in this book may call for ingredients which you haven't often had occasion to use or with which you simply are not familiar. Why goat's milk? And wheat grass -- isn't that for cows?

Green light for goat's milk

As a matter of fact, quite a few recipes in this book call for goat's milk. Many of us have never tasted this dairy product except, perhaps, in the context of feta cheese. You might even wrinkle up your nose at the thought of drinking it, yet fresh, cold goat's milk has a pleasant, creamy flavor. Used in cooking, you won't taste the difference from foods prepared with cow's milk.

But, besides great taste, goat's milk has some important healing properties that cow's milk doesn't. For instance, it's very valuable for people suffering from digestive disturbances, including ulcers. It's much more digestible than cow's milk due to the small size of the fat globules and smaller protein (called casein) particles. Better yet, goat's milk can usually be tolerated by individuals with allergies to cow's milk, as well as by most CFIDS patients and infants with intolerance to formulas containing cow's milk. Such therapeutic benefits are due to a complete absence of alpha S-1 casein, an indigestible protein found in cow's milk. The primary proteins in goat's milk are beta caseins.

If these facts are not entirely convincing, consider that goat's milk contains more potassium, calcium, magnesium, phosphorus, and vitamin A than cow's milk. This is attractive and very important to patients with high protein diets (CFIDS patients), since a high protein intake will generally lead to a deficiency in calcium.

While goat's milk is beginning to enjoy an increased popularity in the US., it is already the leading dairy product in most countries. It's inexpensive to keep goats, and they can thrive in regions that would not support cows. Worldwide, there is no doubt that goat products are more widely consumed than cow products.

Homemade yogurt and cheeses are delicious and easy to prepare using goat's milk. While it takes slightly longer to make than cow's milk yogurt, you can use any yogurt maker to prepare raw or pasteurized goat's milk yogurt. Also, if you haven't yet succumbed to the pleasures of creamy goat and lively feta cheeses, you don't know what you've been missing!

Goat products offer you a new, delicious, and healthy addition to your diet. Let this treasure come into your kitchen!

Wheat grass, the unknown immune booster

Have you juiced your wheat grass today? To more and more people, it's the first question of the morning, and with good reason. City folk don't tend to eat enough leafy green vegetables, yet green foods are the main source of many vitamins and nutrients, essential in protecting and repairing the human body. The most important ingredient of green-leafed vegetables is the magic chlorophyll, a most vital defense against disease.

Wheat grass has an especially high content of chlorophyll. This is a deep green leafy vegetable, reaching its highest content of nutrients in the month of April. Because it does not contain gluten (which causes some people to be allergic to the wheat grain), you don't have to worry about adverse reactions.

The nutritional value of wheat grass is unbelievable! It has a greater protein content (about 25%) than beans and eggs, a higher iron content than spinach, and it contains some 90 different minerals. Its bulking are extremely beneficial during dieting and for cleansing the colon. What a great gift to your body this wheat grass is!

You will find wheat grass especially valuable during the fasting phases described in this book. While some people grow and juice their own wheat grass, most find it more convenient to take it in tablet form. I suggest that most patients take five tablets 15 minutes before meals several times a day. To get the quickest lift, however, an ounce of wheat grass juice is speedily absorbed into by our digestive systems. Wheat grass is a concentrated dream food; may it become a household word in your diet.

Quinoa: Ancient super grain rediscovered

Delicious, high in protein, easy to digest. Sounds too good to be true? Get ready for quinoa (pronounced keen-wa), the sacred grain of the Incas, who used this "mother grain" to build a multinational empire based on their ability to feed all the tribes they conquered. With corn and potatoes, quinoa was considered one of the Incas' three staple foods; extremely hardy and versatile, the plant could grow on rugged land up to 13,000 feet above sea level.

Quinoa's decline began with the arrival of the Spanish conquistadors, who altered agricultural patterns and introduced non-native food crops. A further blow was dealt quinoa by Peruvian authorities themselves in the 1940s with the initiation large-scale wheat imports. But quinoa's popularity is resurging, and not only in South America. Millions of Americans are discovering this nutritious grain, and it is now commercially grown in the Colorado Rockies.

Quinoa is remarkably easy to prepare; it cooks in 15 minutes, making it ideal as a hot breakfast cereal or for a quick lunch dish. It is also wonderful in soups, salads, stuffing, puddings, casseroles, tempeh, breads, pasta, and baked goods. Besides its energizing and strengthening properties (thanks to its high 16% protein content, quinoa has a gourmet versatility and flavor. It is a favorite food for infants and for allergy-prone individuals who appreciate its complete protein make-up and non-allergen properties.

During cooking, quinoa absorbs liquid and expands to four times the original amount. It is high in lysine, methionine, and cystine, three essential amino acids that are found in much lower amounts in other grains. Further, quinoa is richer than other grains in phosphorus, calcium, and iron. So, do yourself a favor. Try quinoa. You'll like it, and so will your friends.

Amaranth: less royal, not less desirable

Amaranth is another newly rediscovered grain. Considered a prime source of energy and vitality by the Aztecs, like quinoa it fell into disfavor after the invasion of the Spaniards. But, as is always the case, you can't keep a good seed down.

Almost a millennium after the Aztecs, we again have the opportunity to discover the beneficial effects of amaranth on our bodies. In fact, quinoa and amaranths are quite similar foods; both contain an average of 16% of protein, with a balance of essential amino acids that is close to ideal. Although no single food can supply all life-sustaining nutrients, quinoa and amaranth come closer than any other food. If this isn't enough, they can be used in all baked goods and are quick and easy to prepare.

Couscous: pearl of the Middle East

Couscous was discovered sometime during the Middle Ages in the Arab-speaking countries of North Africa. After dried pasta, couscous is the most widespread form of semolina (wheat) and, therefore, plays a role in the second phase of our diet plan. Women who can roll semolina into couscous are well-trained and highly-respected artisans in their Arabic homelands. Their skills at making couscous have enormous value; a woman with such talents will be actively courted, her suitors willing to accept a lower dowry to gain this greater prize in marriage.

Unfortunately for those who want to raise their marriage stock, you cannot make couscous from the semolina available here in the US., but the grain is available in cartons in health food stores. It's very easy to prepare (it takes just five minutes to cook) and is a great variant on rice-based meals. If you can boil water, you can make couscous.

Tofu: the "meat of the fields"

In the past, most of Western civilization tended to look upon tofu with a certain disdain. Pale, almost tasteless, and rather odd in texture, this product of soybean curd was completely out of step with the meat-and-potatoes mentality. How things have changed! Today, thanks in large measure to the growing popularity of Chinese or Japanese restaurants, most of us our familiar with this powerful food that the Japanese call "the meat of the fields." The phrase refers to the very high protein content of tofu.

Made from water, carefully selected soybeans (soaked overnight), and a curdling agent made of minerals, what has made tofu so attractive to consumers recently has been its many other fine qualities. It's inexpensive, low in fat, cholesterol-free and preservative-free, and it still has more protein by weight than dairy products and meats.

Today you don't have to go to a Chinese or Japanese market, or even a health food store, to find tofu; due to the increased demand for healthier, simpler diets, even supermarkets now carry this nutritious food. Whether you use it in soups or salads, or stir fry it in your next Chinese meal, tofu will not only please your palate, it will nurture your health.

Lentils: the noble legume

What do Apicius (Roman author of the Western world's first cookbook), Charlemagne of the Holy Roman Empire, and France's Louis XV have in common? However else they were dissimilar, all three had an abiding love for lentils.

Versatile enough to star in many dishes, deeply satisfying, and the easiest legumes to cook (since they require no pre-soaking and cook in about a half an hour), lentils are a dream for every health-minded gastronome. These discus-shaped legumes can play a role at any stage of the meal -- from lentil soups and salads to lentil patties and casseroles.

Lentils are among Earth's most nutritious foods. They're high in protein (second only to soybeans), rich in fiber, high in iron and vitamin B, and contain no cholesterol. Lentils are an almost perfect food.

Prior to preparing lentils, be sure to examine them carefully for bits of stones. Cooking time is about 25 minutes, and eight ounces of lentils will swell to make about four cups of cooked legumes. If you haven't made a delicious pot of lentil soup yet, you don't know what you've been missing!

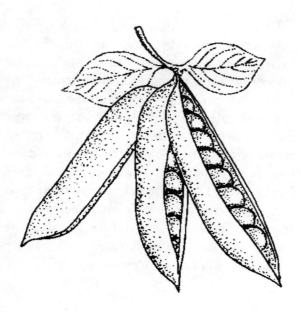

CHAPTER 5

QUESTION TIME

"The doctor of the future will give no medicine but will interest his patients in the care of the human frame, in diet, and in the cause and prevention of disease."

--Thomas Edison

When it comes to healthy eating, knowledge is power. Knowing what you're eating and how it will affect you alleviates the anxiety of continually wondering, worrying, and reacting to the vagaries of trial and error. As in other areas of knowledge, when it comes to food, diet, and health, there are no stupid questions -- except for the one that we fail to ask.

Chapter One answered many of the most obvious food-related questions. This chapter deals with the common concerns of those of us who are setting out on a new, diet-inspired lifestyle on our way to an existence that is full of life. The problems that you will encounter on your individual journey towards better health are universal, and most of the following questions have been repeated again and again by thousands of my patients.

Certainly there are many more questions to be answered, and I would be delighted to hear from you. Becoming a pen pal to others on the way to being full of life is a way of improving my education, and it further stimulates me in my search for the truth.

Can I exercise during fasting?

Among other things, exercise stimulates your circulation and perspiration, both of which are very important when fasting. Because there is an increased release of toxins during fasting, unless you're really feeling too weak to for such activity, moderate exercise is advised to help the body in its detoxification. There are few people who could not do some invigorating walking during fasting. You can set your own pace; there's no competition. Such activity will help alleviate the sluggish feelings of toxin build-up, which can lead to pain and discomfort. Once you have experienced several two-day fasts (and later when you go on to three-day fasts), you'll be pleasantly surprised how much lighter you will feel on the second and third days when moderate exercise is a part of your regimen. I have played in tennis tournaments while fasting, and I've felt light as a feather. However, others may need to preserve their vital energy for the cleansing process, and should take it easy. So, experiment for yourself, and see what level of exercise you're able to do while fasting. Whatever the level, your body will thank you for it.

Why do I become more sensitive as I cleanse my body?

At first glance, it seems odd that one becomes more reactive to food and environmental factors as one gets further along in the program. However, this is natural: as you clean out your body, it begins to react much quicker to all stimuli, and toxic, noxious substances are no exception. It's as if your body is telling you that it will no longer tolerate encounters with poisons; the body is stronger now, and so the strength of its resistance to these poisons is naturally stronger too. Its immediate reaction lets you know you're entering a danger zone. The quicker your immune system reacts, the more grateful you should be. The only thing more important than that reaction is the time you'll need to recuperate from the stimulus. For instance, when I enter a room where there is perfume, I may start sneezing within a minute. But if I stay, after five minutes I stop sneezing because my immune system is able to pull me out of this hyper-reactivity. Those whose immune systems might be more impaired might not feel well for rest of the day, or longer. As you get cleaner and stronger, your reaction time gets shorter, reflecting the increased strength of your immune system. In fact, not reacting to the perfume can be a sign of a suppressed immune system -- that it is too fatigued or "lazy" to warn you. Another example: it is very common that, on this improved diet, tolerance for alcohol will go down significantly. Whereas in the past you could drink two glasses of wine, now you get drunk after half a glass. When this happens, don't say, "Poor me! I can't drink anymore!" Instead, be grateful that your body is awakening to the toxicity in this world.

I cheated a few times on my program; did I lose everything I've gained so far?

No. This happens to all of us, so don't let it devastate you. Simply realize that, no, you didn't lose everything you've gained, but you should learn from this little incident. Did it taste as good as you thought it would be? Was it truly satisfying, and how long did the satisfaction last? What were your immediate reactions after eating or drinking this forbidden fruit? Did you experience muscle pains, headaches, constipation, or other symptoms? The next time you're being seduced by those goodies, remember how this felt. Maybe you'll conclude that it isn't worth it!

Why can my friends eat whatever they want without being affected by it?

This is what we call a "fata morgana" or dream picture. Your friends, ostensibly not affected by junk food, don't react because their bodies are "numb" all the time. Their real energy level (not the one produced by coffee and sugar) is so low that a little more drop will not be felt. Your friends think that fatigue, hang-overs, headaches, and bloating are just part of normal life. If they don't clean up their acts, however, they'll never know the "other world." Amazingly enough, their skin always seems to look better than yours. We should remember that the rougher the outsides or exterior (skin) of our body looks, the better our interior or organs function. It is the skin's job to help you expelling toxins.

I don't like legumes or beans. Am I doing myself harm by not eating them?

We've spoken about lentils in particular, however legumes in general are rich in the B vitamins, vitamins A and E, and potassium, calcium, phosphorus, and iron. While other beans, such as pintos, need to be combined with cheese to form a complete protein, the soybean is alone in the legume world in offering all the amino acids needed by the body to synthesize protein. This wonder bean also contains twice as much calcium and thiamin as other beans. This becomes important for vegetarians or patients on a rich protein diet: Enough calcium can be gotten by eating soybeans and soy products. Other high sources of calcium are tofu, kale, cheddar goat's cheese, goat's milk and goat's yogurt, collard greens, brewer's yeast, leafy green vegetables, nuts, and seeds. It is very important to cook soybeans very well to destroy an enzyme that otherwise retards the digestion of protein and to avoid intestinal gas. Legumes, though not complete proteins on their own, supply half over the world with a major part of its protein, but they must be combined with other forms of protein to form complete proteins. So eat more legumes; they're some of the highest quality plant protein available!

I have a wheat allergy, and I have difficulties grain products that are not wheat related. Do I have to do all my own baking now?

You might know that wheat is the most widely-cultivated grain and food crop. No surprise, therefore, that many people become allergic or sensitive to it. So the search is on for substitutes. Is durum semolina okay? What about the vegetable pastas? Bulgur? Triticale? Milo? Buckwheat? Durum Semolina is just another name for wheat, and even so-called vegetable pastas (spinach, beet, etc.) are usually 90% wheat, so they're not good substitutes for wheat allergies. Bulgur is called the "rice of the Middle East," but it, too, is actually a cracked wheat product. Triticale, one of the newcomers, is a cross between rye and wheat, while milo, or sorghum, resembles corn botanically. Buckwheat, despite its name, is more closely related to rhubarb and is considerably more nourishing than other grains; it's actually the dried seeds of a plant which can be ground into a satisfactory flour. So buckwheat and milo are "in," triticale and bulgur are "out."

"All-purpose" flour is a combination of hard and soft wheat, used for breads and cakes. It should be low on your list! Menomin is an Indian name for wild rice, for centuries harvested by hand. According to an old Indian tradition, one person guides the boat, another person knocks the rice off the stalks into a basket. Graham flour is nothing but soft whole wheat flour, named after the 19th century health food advocate, Sylvester Graham.

I suffer from constipation, and my doctor tells me to eat more fiber. What is dietary fiber, and how does it work?

Dietary fiber is plant material that is largely indigestible and therefore unabsorbed by the body. There are two varieties: soluble and insoluble. Soluble fibers, present in oatmeal and legumes, are gummy and help block the absorption of fats, which helps lower the body's cholesterol levels. Insoluble fibers, so-called because they won't break down in water, absorb water in the digestive tract, while extracting and expelling waste material. Much attention was paid to President Reagan's surgery for a colon polyp, increasing the awareness of the need for diets high in insoluble fibers (apple peel, for example). Fiber-rich foods are virtually fat-free and, since they also make it more difficult for the body to absorb fat, they are ideal allies for dieters. In fact, many so-called wonder pills contain mostly dietary fiber. While the ideal fiber intake is about 35 to 40 grams daily, Americans typically average only about 10 to 20 grams. Other excellent sources of dietary fiber are bran cereals, baked beans, dried figs, raw apples, and whole-wheat bread. In general, the less refined the food is, the more fiber it has.

I want to lose weight fast, so I skip breakfast. Is this a good idea?

Five thousand years ago, the Chinese would have had you killed for such a crime! Breakfast (breaking the fast) is the most important meal of the day. The digestive organs (spleen-pancreas and stomach) have their "working hours" (according to the Chinese clock) from 7 a.m. until 11 a.m. So don't get them into the habit of not waking them up for work! They'll just get lazy. And if you inundate them with a big meal at night, they won't be able to respond to this enormous stimulus. Skipping breakfast will have no significant effect on weight loss. On the contrary, in recent years people have begun to skip breakfast more and more often, and our children pay the consequences in poor attitudes towards school work, a tendency to be overweight, and a decreased pattern of exercise. Skip breakfast, and you'll be starting out on the wrong foot!

My cholesterol level is too high; what should I do about it?

Not all cholesterol is bad. (See Chapter One, Principle 6: Know Your Fats.) In fact, the human body needs cholesterol to function -- but it generally produces enough on its own. Cholesterol is manufactured mainly in the liver and is found in every cell of the body. It is especially critical for proper functioning of the brain and is found in abundance in the spinal cord and nerves as well as the brain. Further, the fat-soluble vitamins A, D, E, and K require cholesterol to properly carry out their functions. Your HDL or High Density Lipoprotein cholesterol is your good cholesterol (nl. between 40-90). The higher your count is the <u>better</u>. The LDL or low Density Lipoprotein is the "bad" guy (nl. between 60-180). The lower your count is the better. Keep in mind that a <u>total</u> cholesterol count does not give you correct information. What you want to know is the LDL-HDL Risk Ratio since this will give you the real risk factor of heart disease.

Foods to avoid are saturated fats, hydrogenated fats (peanut butter, margarine, and shortening), and fat from animal products (i.e., meat, poultry, eggs, fish, milk, butter, and cheese). I do, however, believe that eggs and butter have gotten their bad reputations rather unjustly. Other sources of increased cholesterol are smoking, emotional upheaval, and stress while exercise will decrease these levels.

When you will follow the good food list (Chapter One) on page 36, you'll be pleasantly surprised that your cholesterol count will decrease despite eating eggs and butter, even on a daily basis. Sugar, junk food, fatty meats, and preservatives are all toxic to your liver. Therefore the liver will produce a higher amount of LDL. It is unfortunate that more studies have not been done to prove this, but thus far, in my daily practice, I definitely see the relationship between sugar intake and LDL increase.

I am trying to improve my health by eating better. What role do minerals play?

Minerals are vital to human health. Some minerals are called "essential" because they're required for the body to function; others are called trace minerals, which are also believed necessary for general health and also for strengthening the body's reserves in preparation for one of life's little traumas.

One key essential mineral is potassium, which is found chiefly in bananas, dried peas and beans, dried fruits (like apricots and peaches), and in lesser degrees in most other foods, including fish and meat.

Chlorine (or chloride) is another vital mineral; it is required for the production of the digestive juices, and can be found in sea salt, tomatoes, and leafy vegetables.

Magnesium, found in egg yolks, nuts, dark green vegetables, and goat's milk, performs many functions. It is important for the formation of bones, metabolism of calcium, functioning of the muscles, and the regulation of the nervous system.

Phosphorus is another important mineral. To be effective, it needs to be consumed in a ratio of three-to-one with calcium; otherwise, both become less effective. Phosphorus plays a role in the strengthening of bones and teeth, in the functioning of brain cells, and in the maintenance of the proper acid-alkaline blood balance. Legumes -- especially soybeans, milk, and meats -- are rich in phosphorus.

Copper is another mineral essential to nutrition. It is required for the utilization of iron in the body and maintains normal skin and hair coloring. Copper is found in mushrooms, molasses, and organ meats.

Reading the above list of minerals and their functions, you might notice that some of the sources are not allowed according to this diet plan. Therefore, especially in the first phase (i.e., milk, molasses, mushrooms, etc.), it is wise to add a multimineral supplement to your diet. This is equally important for young children, pregnant women, post-operative patients (trace minerals as well), and for anyone who does not, as a rule, eat a well-balanced diet.

Now that I've decided to eat healthier, I get confused by all the different things labeled as "health food."

There is little doubt that the food industry has purposely tried to confuse people with misleading labels. However new laws, imposed by the FDA on the food industry in 1993, will hopefully help the consumer to zigzag through the jungle of food information. While you are perhaps already familiar with soybean and triticale products, other products make you wonder if they're really healthy, or natural, or neither?

One of these is brewer's yeast. Yeast has gotten a bad rap, but brewer's yeast should get exempted from this. Brewer's yeast is an excellent source of selenium and B vitamins; mixed with juices or used in cooking, it also supplies amino acids, calcium, trace minerals, and magnesium.

Bulgur? This is essentially wheat that has been parboiled. It resembles and cooks like rice. The Middle East dish, "tabouli," is a favorite recipe that uses bulgur.

Miso? It is made from soybeans, salt, and water; it's used to enhance a variety of foods, including soups and sauces. Miso and tofu are allowed in the Phase 2 of the diet, not in the Phase 1, because they are manufactured in a fermentation process.

What about carob? Carob is good news for all of us chocolate addicts. It is an excellent substitute for cocoa and chocolate, and it can be used in cakes, cookies, and muffins with a but less guilt. Blackstrap molasses on the other hand is a by-product of refining sugar cane or sugar beets. Black strap molasses isn't allowed during Phase 1 because it is too concentrated in sweet flavor.

As for you peanut butter lovers, choose tahini or sesame butter instead. While the former typically carries too much mold, the latter is high in protein. Unfortunately, they're high in fat, too, as with other nut butters, you should use them sparingly because of their high calorie content.

Swiss muesli is an untoasted cereal made from various unroasted grains mixed with dried fruits (i.e., oats and apples). Because this is a more complicated combination, don't try it in the first four weeks of your improved diet. Granola is similar, although the grains are toasted.

What can I do for my children?

Common sense tells us that the same rules that apply to the health of adults should be applied to the health of children. It amazes me when parents ask, "How can I not give my kids junk food? It's part of our culture, and they love it so much!" My reply: "If you really love them, how can you give it to them."

Naturally, having junk food on hand for the kids is the perfect excuse for the adult to succumb as well. But be aware that more and more studies are showing that there is a direct relationship between junk food, aggressive behavior, and poor academic performance. Further, according to a Yale University study, the chances are about one in four that a childhood bully will have a criminal record by age 30.

While you're at it, put a limit on TV watching. Your child will have a greatly increased tendency to become overweight because of the combination of passivity and increased snacking. If you love your kids, make a change today! Replace junk snacks with healthy snacks, and replace television with real-life experiences.

I am confused about vitamin supplements. Can they really do anything for me?

I've already suggested certain supplements to complement the phases of this Full of Life diet. While you want to be sure that you, indeed, absorb all the vitamins you take in, it is equally important that you don't lose sight of the reasons you're taking certain supplements in the first place. Too often, patients take 50 pills a day and haven't the foggiest why. So, let's review some of the vitamins and how they can assist you on the road to being Full of Life.

Dry skin is one inevitable consequence of an improved diet. The liver has a hard time processing the increased amount of toxins, therefore your skin has to play a more active role in the elimination process. Vitamin A is well known as an ally in maintaining or restoring good night vision, but it can also help heal your dry, scaly skin. Rather than the usual vitamin A, take the pro-vitamin A, beta carotene. This adds an extra safeguard, since beta carotene is only converted to vitamin A as needed, within six hours of its consumption. Take beta carotene (25,000 I.U) twice a day. The best food sources for beta carotene are sweet potatoes, peaches, apricots, kale, spinach, collards, and carrots.

Many of us suffer from drug toxicity and environmental overloads; this is expressed through our sensitivities. Vitamin E (400 I.U/daily) together with selenium (100 mcg/daily) will come to your aid. Vitamin E is also a strong ally in fighting cystic breast disease, heart dysfunction, and circulation disturbances. I give vitamin E an "A."

Going through major health changes (even cleansing) is stressful, and there's nothing better than vitamin B complex to keep you in balance. Make sure you take a product that is yeast-free; if this is not mentioned on the label, it isn't! Take a tablet in the morning and at noon. Avoid vitamin B complex in the evening, or you'll have a hard time falling asleep!

Can I ever return to milk products once I reach the "Full of Life" phase?

Normally you can. However, many people experience a lactose intolerance -- they're unable to properly break down and digest this sugar due to a lack of the enzyme, lactase. If such is the case for you, it would be good to take small amounts of a lactobacillus cultured on milk. This way you'll be able to introduce small amounts of lactase into your system since this is part of the lactobacillus culture. If you don't like goat's milk after six months on the diet, you can try introducing a "lactate" milk (i.e., Lactaid), which contains small amounts of lactase.

I can give up almost anything, but not my morning coffee!

This should tell you how addicted you are to this "medication." It looks like you can't make it to work without getting a lick from the coffee whip! Unfortunately, as Hahnemann, the father of Homeopathy and the last medical genius stated 200 years ago, this will only lead to an increased intake as time goes on. Don't bother telling me that you never have constipation until you stop drinking coffee. Quitting coffee isn't easy and it will inevitably lead to withdrawal symptoms like headaches, fatigue, muscle and joint pains, and so on. This can be helped by the homeopathic remedy Chamomilla 30C, three pellets three times a day. But give it up, you must, if you ever want to be full of life! You can help yourself "cut the cord" with chicory or bachelor buttons, whose roots can be roasted and brewed to create a palatable coffee substitute. You can also achieve the same result with dandelion root. Any of these are also rich in vitamin A.

I hate having dark circles under my eyes. Is there anything I can do?

Unfortunately, switching from a junk diet to a healthy diet might temporarily cause those dreaded dark marks. According to Chinese medicine, these are caused by the workings of the kidneys and the adrenal cortex, reflecting the stress your body is under. So, no creams or wonder pills are going to help you with this. In the long run, however, an improved diet, proper rest, and excellent elimination will do much to improve your overall looks as well the area under the eyes. In the meantime, use diuretic teas (i.e., parsley tea and cranberry root) and reduce any puffiness by applying a chilled black tea bag to the eye area (the tannin in the tea is astringent).

What can I do about these hard, painful boils?

As long as you understand that these boils are an expression of your cleansing program, you won't make the mistake of trying to apply cortisone creams, which will do nothing for the problem except create another imbalance by making your skin thinner, possibly leading to "cortisone acne." Ordinarily, these boils melt away as time goes on. Don't let anyone inject cortisone into them! This would only push your toxins back into your body where they will do more harm to the organs. (See suppression in *Human Condition: Critical*). However, certain herbal infusions (taken internally or applied externally) can be helpful. Burdock especially has good cleansing capacities. You might want to fill your own capsules, mixing it with yellow dock and ginseng roots. Try two capsules, three times a day. Also the homeopathic remedies Hepar Sulph. or Silica 30C will assist you in melting these boils down without side-effects. Take one pellet in 4 oz. of water, stir well and take one tsp. three times a day.

By cutting out dairy products, I'm afraid I'll get osteoporosis.

Osteoporosis is not just another inevitable result of growing old. With foresight and adequate supplemental intake, you can lessen your chances of developing osteoporosis. You might think that an increased protein intake would draw calcium from your tissues and, combined with a decreased intake of dairy products, put you at greater risk of osteoporosis. Not entirely true. As mentioned earlier, there are many foods that contain more calcium than you thought (goat products, seeds, nuts, broccoli, etc.). Other excellent food calcium sources are kale and dark, leafy vegetables. Sardines with bones and canned salmon with bones, are two other sources. And don't forget: Exercise increases bone growth! A daily 20-minute walk can do the job. Remember also that some foods are calcium blockers; oxalic acid, a substance present in spinach, beet greens, and rhubarb is one of those. Avoid excessive amounts of phosphorus, too, since it will increase the body's need for calcium. Finally, eliminate the largest known risk factors for osteoporosis: coffee, alcohol, and tobacco! An excellent homeopathic remedy to avoid osteoporosis is Calc. Phos. 6C, three pellets twice a day. This can be taken for months at the time.

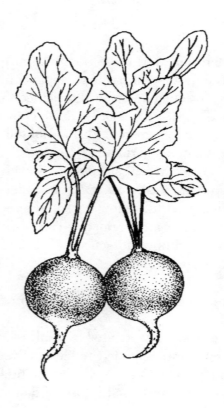

CHAPTER SIX

SALADS AND DRESSINGS

Super Shrimp Salad

1 cup cooked shrimp
1 stalk celery, with leaves
   sliced
2 tablespoons chopped green
   onion
1/2 head lettuce, cleaned & coarsely
   torn into large bite-size pieces
   (substitute: spinach)

1 medium tomato
1/2 green pepper, chopped
1/2 cucumber, chopped
2 tablespoons fresh
parsley, minced

In a large salad bowl mix together the shrimp and all the vegetables. Serve at once.
Serves 4-6.

✳

Macaroni & Tuna Salad

2 cups cooked elbow macaroni
(quinoa)
1 cup celery, finely chopped
2 tablespoons onion, finely
1/4 cup carrot, cleaned/grated

1/4 cup plain yogurt
1 cup fresh peas, lightly steamed
1/4 cup mayonnaise
dash paprika
1 small can tuna, well drained

Mix cooked macaroni, celery, onion, carrot and tuna in a large bowl. In a separate bowl,
stir yogurt (goat) and mayonnaise together to make a dressing. Fold the dressing through
the macaroni mixture until it is well coated. Garnish with paprika, cover, and chill in the
refrigerator for about 2 hours before serving.
Yields 4-6 servings.

Easy Veggie-Rice Salad

1 stalk celery	1/2 teaspoon cumin powder
1 medium zucchini	1/4 teaspoon paprika
2 medium tomatoes, seeded	1 teaspoon Dijon mustard
2 cups cooked brown rice	3 tablespoons lemon juice

Chop the celery, zucchini and tomatoes finely --- about rice-grain size. A food processor may be used. Mix together the cumin, paprika, mustard and lemon juice. Toss all ingredients together. Taste for seasoning.

Yields 4 servings.

✳

Beet Salad

3 cups cooked, sliced beets, and chilled	1/4 cup chopped onion
2 hard-cooked eggs, chopped	4 lettuce cups (or spinach)
	sprigs of fresh parsley

Mix sliced beets, chopped eggs and onion together in a mixing bowl. Divide salad mixture into four portions and spoon each portion into a lettuce cup. Garnish with parsley and serve.

Serves 3 persons.

✳

Arabian Beet Salad

5 large beets	1/4 lemon juice
2 cloves garlic	1/4 olive oil
1 1/2 teaspoon sea salt	1/2 teaspoon pepper
1/4 cup fresh chives, finely chopped	
2 tablespoons fresh coriander, finely chopped	

Boil the beets until they are thoroughly cooked. Peel, dice into small pieces and place in salad bowl. Mash garlic with sea salt, then add to the beets. Add pepper, coriander, chives, olive oil and lemon juice, gently mix. Sprinkle with parsley. Chill before serving.

Yields 4-6 servings.

Orange and Radish Salad (Full of Life phase)

6 seedless oranges, peeled
1/2 cup lemon juice
3 tablespoons rice syrup
1/4 teaspoon cinnamon

1 cup red radishes, soaked
in water for 1 hour,
coarsely grated

OPTIONAL:
1/8 teaspoon orange blossom water

Section oranges into salad bowl, set aside. In another bowl place lemon juice, orange blossom water, rice syrup and salt, stir until rice syrup and salt are dissolved. Add lemon solution and radishes to oranges and toss gently, sprinkle with cinnamon and serve.
NOTE:

> The salad must be served immediately. If allowed to stand for a long period of time, the taste will change. Yields 4-6 servings.
> • Persons with digestive problems should avoid this recipe (fruit with veggies)

Vegetable Salad

1 cup fresh green peas, cooked
1 cup fresh green beans, cooked
4 tablespoons plain yogurt,
  goats
4 tablespoons olive oil
3 tablespoons chopped parsley

1/2 teaspoon sea salt
1/2 teaspoon pepper
3 tomatoes, diced
3 tablespoons lemon juice
1 large beet, cooked,
peeled and sliced thin

In a salad bowl mix the green beans, peas, tomatoes, yogurt. olive oil, tomatoes and lemon juice. Sprinkle sea salt/pepper, toss. Decorate with beets and parsley, chill and serve.

Yields 4-6 servings.

Cheese Salad

1 1/2 cups onion, finely sliced
1 1/2 cups cabbage, finely
  sliced
1 cup carrots, finely shredded
1 1/2 cups tomatoes, chopped
  into large pieces

1/4 cup lemon juice
1/4 cup olive juice
 2 teaspoons sea salt
1/2 teaspoon pepper
1 clove garlic, crushed
1/2 cup white cheese,
  grated (goat)

Place onion, cabbage, carrots and tomatoes in bowl, mix well. In a small bowl, mix lemon juice, olive oil, sea salt, pepper and garlic, pour over the vegetables and toss. Sprinkle cheese over salad and serve.

    Yields 4-6 servings.

✳

Tomato Salad

3 medium sized tomatoes,
  chopped into small pieces
1 medium size cucumber,
  chopped into small pieces
1 large sweet pepper, chopped
1/2 bunch parsley, finely
  chopped
1/2 bunch green onions. finely
  chopped

juice of 2 lemons
1 1/2 teaspoon sea salt
1/2 teaspoon pepper
6 red radishes, chopped
1/4 cup white cheese
1 clove garlic, crushed
1/4 cup virgin olive oil
2 tablespoons fresh mint chopped

Mix all ingredients, except the cheese, and allow to marinate for 10 minutes. Sprinkle the cheese pieces evenly over the top and serve.

    Yields 4-6 servings.

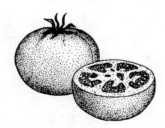

Eggplant Salad

1 large eggplant
2 teaspoons sea salt
2 cloves garlic
1/2 small tomato, diced into small pieces

3 tablespoons virgin olive oil
1/3 cup sesame tahini
1/3 cup fresh lemon juice

OPTIONAL:

1 tablespoon pomegranate seeds
1 tablespoon fried pine nuts
a few parsley sprigs

Place eggplant in a pan. Bake in 425 degree oven turning frequently until well cooked. Allow to cool, remove and discard skin, mash pulp well and set aside. Mash the garlic with 1 tea-spoon salt, add 1 teaspoon lemon juice and mix until smooth, add to eggplant. Place remaining lemon juice and tahini in blender for a few moments, add to eggplant. Stir in remaining sea salt, spread on a platter. Sprinkle with the olive oil and garnish with parsley, pomegranate seeds, pine nuts and tomato pieces.

Yields 4-6 servings.

✻

Tropical Fruit Salad

2 bananas
2 kiwi fruit

1 cup plain yogurt, goats
1 papaya

Peel and slice the bananas into the serving bowl. Peel kiwi and cut it into thin slices on the width and add to bowl. Next, peel, seed, and cube papaya and place with the other fruits. Toss all together and then stir in yogurt (goats). May be served on a bed of lettuce or alfalfa sprouts.

Serves 3.

VARIATIONS:

Replace all or part of the papaya with peeled and cubed mango.

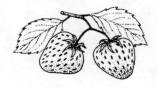

Artichoke Pasta Salad

4 cups white and green
   spiral pasta, cooked
1 medium carrot, chopped
parsley for garnish

1 jar marinated artichoke
   hearts, drained
1/3-1 cup favorite dressing

Cook pasta according to package directions. Drain, rinse and set aside. Mix together carrot and artichoke hearts. Add pasta and mix everything thoroughly. Add your favorite dressing and mix it thoroughly through other ingredients. Garnish with sprigs of crisp parsley. Refrigerate for several hours before serving.
    Serves 4.

✳

Pasta Salad with Peas and Celery

1/2 cup cooked pasta
1/2 cup cooked peas,

1 scallion, chopped
1/4 cup celery, chopped

Combine all ingredients and top with favorite dressing.
    Serves 2.

✳

Zucchini-Spinach Salad

1 small bunch scallions
   about 5 or 6
2 small or 1 medium zucchini
1 1/2 cups torn spinach

1 cup sliced celery hearts
1 cup torn leaf lettuce
1 large tomato, chopped

Wash scallions and chop fine. Wash zucchini and cut off stem end. Do not peel. Slice zucchini very thin. If zucchini is medium sized, cut the slices in half. Mix scallions, zucchini, celery, greens and tomato in large salad bowl. Serve with favorite dressing.
    Serves 2.

Beetroot Salad

2 cups cooked beets, sliced
   thinly
1 small onion, minced
pinch cayenne

1/2 teaspoon sea salt
1/2 teaspoon garam masala
2 tablespoons lemon juice

Separately combine, salt, garam masala, lemon juice and cayenne. Add beets and onion. Chill and serve garnished with yogurt (goats).
> *Yields 4 servings.*

Halibut Salad

1 tablespoon chopped onion
mayonnaise
1 cucumber, peeled/cubed
lettuce

1/4 teaspoon pepper
3 cups cold cooked halibut
1 teaspoon sea salt

The halibut should have been cooked in very salty water - at least 2 teaspoons of salt to each quart of water. Flake the halibut in rather large pieces. Moisten with French dressing and chill thoroughly. Mix the halibut, cucumber, onion, sea salt and pepper with sufficient mayonnaise to hold the ingredients together. The mayonnaise may be thinned with a little cream. Serve on crisp lettuce leaves on a large platter.
> *Serves 8.*

Shrimp Salad

8 tender stalks, celery with
   leaves
1 orange cut into wedges
mayonnaise

1/2 cups cleaned cooked
   shrimp
2 carrots, cut into strips

Divide a chop plate into 4 sections with celery stalks. Place shrimp, orange wedges and carrots in each section. Serve mayonnaise in bowl in center.
> *Serves 4.*

Green Bean Salad Bowl

3 cups cooked green beans
1/3 cup French dressing
1/2 cup sliced radishes

1 small onion, minced
lettuce leaves

Combine beans, radishes and onion with French dressing. Chill for 1 hour. Drain and toss in salad bowl. Garnish with lettuce.
  Serves 6.

Egg and Onion Salad Bowl

1 head lettuce
8 hard-cooked eggs
1/3 cup grated sharp cheese
  (goats)

4 medium onions
1 tablespoon minced parsley
lemon French dressing

Shred lettuce and toss with dressing. Arrange alternate layers of sliced onions and eggs over lettuce in salad bowl. Moisten with additional dressing, sprinkle with cheese and garnish with parsley.
  Serves 6.

Spring Salad Bowl

2 cups cooked peas
6 cooked cauliflowers
2 cups cooked green beans
2 tomatoes, peeled/sliced

1 head lettuce
watercress
French or Roquefort dressing

Marinate vegetables separately in French dressing and chill for 1 hour. Line salad bowl with outside leaves of lettuce and place 4 lettuce cups around center of bowl. Fill each with one of the vegetables and garnish center of bowl with watercress.
  Yields 6 servings.

Salad Bowl of Vegetables Julienne

1 small cucumber, pared
1 cup shredded cooked carrots
1 cup shredded cooked green
   beans

olive oil
French Dressing
lettuce

Cut cucumber into long slender strips, add beans and carrots and marinate in dressing. Shred lettuce into large pieces and toss in salad bowl with olive oil Drain marinated vegetables and arrange in center of bowl.

Serves 6.

✳

Buffet Potato Salad

2 cups cold, cubed, cooked
diced potatoes
2 small onions, diced
1 cup cold cooked peas

1 green pepper,
1 cup mayonnaise
1/2 teaspoon sea salt
4 hard-cooked eggs, diced

Combine potatoes, peas, eggs, onions, green pepper and sea salt. Mix with mayonnaise. Chill thoroughly and serve on lettuce.

Serves 4 to 6.

✳

Tomato Cauliflower Salad

1/2 head cauliflower
watercress

3 tomatoes, peeled and chilled
Roquefort dressing

Cut each tomato crosswise into halves. Soak cauliflowers in salted water for 45 minutes. Separate into small flowerets. Arrange 1 tomato half on watercress on each plate, top with cauliflowerets and serve with dressing.

Serves 6.

Minted Lamb Salad

2 cups thin small slices cold cooked lamb 2 cups sliced cooked potatoes
mint   French dressing
lettuce hearts   1/4 teaspoon sea salt

Combine lamb and potatoes; add sea salt and marinate in dressing for 1 hour. Drain.
Toss lettuce hearts with dressing in salad bow, heap lamb and potato salad on lettuce and
garnish with sprigs of mint.
   Serves 6.

✳

Avocado Filled with Salmon

2 avocados   1 cup diced celery
lemon juice   1 cup flaked salmon
sea salt   1/2 cup mayonnaise

Cut avocados lengthwise into halves, remove seeds and sprinkle cut portion with lemon
juice and sea salt. Combine celery and salmon with mayonnaise to moisten. Fill centers
of avocados.
   Serves 4.
VARIATIONS:
        Use 1 cup crab meat, lobster, or shrimp instead of salmon.

✳

Crab-Flake Salad

2 cups crab flakes, fresh   1 cup mayonnaise
   cooked or canned   1/4 teaspoon sea salt
2 tablespoons lemon juice   salad greens
1 cup celery, diced   2 teaspoons grated onion

Combine all ingredients. Serve in a bowl garnished with salad greens or in lettuce cups as
individual servings.
   Serves 4.

Romaine and Shrimp Salad

12 stalks cooked asparagus
12 slices hard-cooked egg
4 green pepper rings
mayonnaise

12 large cooked shrimp
4 long, 4 short leaves
romaine

Arrange 3 large stalks asparagus, topped with 3 slices of egg and 3 shrimp on each long romaine leaf. Beside it, on the shorter leaf place a pepper ring filled with mayonnaise.
Serves 4.

✳

Molded Cucumber Salad

1 cucumber, pared/diced
1/2 teaspoon sea salt
2 teaspoons unflavored gelatin

1/2 teaspoon lemon juice
1/4 cup cold water
1 cup cream, whipped

Combine cucumber, sea salt and lemon juice. Soak gelatin in cold water 5 minutes; dissolve over hot water and mix thoroughly with whipped cream. Add cucumber mixture and pour into molds. Chill.
Yields 4 servings.

✳

Cranberry Ring Salad

2 cups cranberries
1 1/2 cups cold water
1 tablespoon unflavored gelatin
lettuce

3/4 cup diced celery
1 cup rice syrup
1/2 cup chopped nuts
mayonnaise

Wash cranberries, add 1 cup cold water. Cook until tender. Add rice syrup and cook for 5 minutes. Soften gelatin in 1/2 cup cold water, dissolve in hot cranberries. Chill until mixture begins to thicken. Add nuts and celery. Mix thoroughly. Pour into oiled ring mold. Chill until firm. Unfold and place on large salad plate. Place light lettuce around salad, arrange shrimp in center or serve on a bed of letter on individual plates and garnish with mayonnaise.
Serves 8.

Appetizer Salad

1 1/2 cups thin slices carrots
1 hard-cooked egg, sliced
watercress or lettuce

1 small cucumber
pearl onion
French dressing

Place carrot slices in ice water for 1 hour until crisp. Score the pared cucumber lengthwise with a fork, cut into thin slices and chill. Arrange carrot and cucumber slices on watercress (or lettuce), place a ring of egg white in center of each salad and sprinkle with sieved yolk. Serve with French dressing.
   Serves 6.

Molded Tuna Salad

1 (7 ounce) can tuna
1 hard-cooked egg, chopped
1/2 tablespoon minced onion
lettuce

1/2 tablespoon unflavored
   gelatin
1 cup mayonnaise
1/8 cup cold water

Mince tuna, hard-cooked egg and onion. Soften gelatin in cold water 5 minutes, dissolve over hot water and add to mayonnaise gradually, stirring constantly. Fold into tuna mixture. Turn unto mold and chill until firm. Unmold on lettuce.
   Serves 2.

Salad with Tuna & Feta

4 cups leaf lettuce
16 sweet onion rings
1 can water packed tuna chunks

1 cup Feta cheese (sheep)
   crumbled

Toss lettuce with Lemon Dressing (see below). Arrange on plate and arrange olives and tuna around edges. Garnish with onion rings and Feta cheese.
   Serves 4.

Lemon Dressing (Full of Life Phase)

1 clove garlic, minced
generous dash dried oregano
1/4 cup apple juice

sea salt/pepper to taste
1/3 cup fresh lemon juice
1/4 cup safflower oil

Combine all ingredients and beat or shake together. Makes about 1 cup dressing.

SEAFOOD, VEGETABLE, SALAD, FRUIT DRESSINGS, & SPREADS

Avocado Salad Dressing

2 very ripe avocados
1 tablespoon grated onion

sea salt to taste
pinch garlic

Put the above ingredients in blender and serve on salads or chilled veggies.

✳

Beet Salad Dressing

4 medium-size beets
1/4 cup beet liquid
6 tablespoons mayonnaise

2 tablespoons lemon juice
1 tablespoon minced onion
1 tablespoon minced garlic

Cook beets in water to cover until tender. Drain and reserve 1/4 cup beet liquid. Peel and quarter beets. Combine all ingredients in blender and process until smooth.
Yields approx. 2 cups.

Emerald Dressing
(seafoods or green salads)

1 cup corn oil

1/3 cup fresh lemon juice

1 cup chopped green pepper

1 teaspoon dill

1/2 teaspoon sea salt

1/4 cup chopped parsley

1/4 cup chopped onion

Combine all ingredients in blender. Process for about 3 minutes.
Yields 1 1/2 cups.

✳

Yogurt Salad Dressing

3/4 cup yogurt (goat)

2 tablespoons fresh lemon juice

1 teaspoon prepared mustard

1/2 teaspoon kelp powder

1 onion, grated

1 teaspoon basil

1/2 teaspoon sea salt

1/8 teaspoon pepper

1 clove garlic, minced

Combine all ingredients and mix well. Allow to stand in refrigerator for at least 20 minutes before serving.
Yields approx. 1 1/4 cups.

✳

Spicy Yogurt Dressing (Full of Life)
(fruit salads)

1 cup yogurt (goat)

3 tablespoons apple juice

1/4 teaspoon finely grated
   lemon rind

1/4 teaspoon cinnamon

pinch nutmeg

1 tablespoon rice syrup

Mix all ingredients thoroughly and chill until ready to use.
Yields 1 1/4 cups.

Avocado Dressing
(serve as a spread or fruit dressing)

2 ripe avocados
1/4 cup chopped sunflower
  seeds

1/4 cup wheat germ
1 tablespoon lemon juice

Peel and pit the avocados. Mash with a fork until smooth. Add wheat germ, lemon juice and sunflower seeds. Mix until well combined.
  Yields 1 1/2 cups.

✳

Sweet French Dressing

1/2 cup salad oil
1/2 cup fresh lemon juice

2 tablespoons rice syrup
dash cayenne red pepper

Shake all ingredients in tightly covered jar.
  Yields 1 cup.

✳

French Dressing

1 cup olive oil
1/2 teaspoon sea salt
1/4 teaspoon white pepper

1/4 cup lemon juice
few grains cayenne
2 cups chopped parsley

Combine and beat thoroughly before using.
  Makes 1 1/4 cups.
VARIATIONS using 1 cup French Dressing as a foundation...
  Garlic - Rub bowl with crushed clove garlic
  Chive - Add 1 tablespoon chopped chives, minced shallot or onion.
  Cucumber - Add 3 tablespoons grated cucumber and 1 tablespoon chopped
       chives.

Lemon French Dressing

1/2 cup olive oil
1/2 cup lemon juice
Few grains cayenne
1/2 teaspoon sea salt
2 tablespoons rice syrup

Combine all ingredients and shake well before using. Makes 1 cup.
VARIATIONS with 1 cup Lemon French Dressing...
Lime: Use 1/4 cup lime juice instead of 1/4 cup lemon juice.
Mint: Add 2 tablespoons chopped mint.

✻

Chili Dressing

1/2 cup mayonnaise
1/4 cup chili sauce (mild)
1 teaspoon minced green pepper

Mix well and chill.

✻

Garlic Dressing

3 cups olive oil
1/2 cup chopped parsley
5 sliced garlic cloves
1 tablespoon kelp

Blend or mix in a bottle. Let marinate for 1/2 day.

✻

Garlic Yogurt Dressing

2 cloves garlic, chopped
1 leafy stalk celery, chopped
1 cup yogurt (goat)
1 leafy stalk celery, chopped
2 scallions, chopped
1/3 cup parsley, chopped
1 Tbs. Worcestershire sauce
1/4 cup onion, chopped

Mix all ingredients in blender and blend until smooth.

Light and Lemony Dressing
(green salads)

1/3 cup fresh lemon juice	2/3 cup vegetable oil
(2 lemons)	sea salt/pepper to taste
1 garlic clove, minced	scallion, chopped

Squeeze juice from lemons. Combine lemon juice and vegetable oil in small saucepan. Heat for one minute; add garlic. Remove from heat and stir in scallion. Season with sea salt/pepper.

Yields 1 cup.

✳

Basic Blender Mayonnaise

1 egg, room temperature	1 teaspoon Dijon mustard
1/2 to 3/4 cup olive oil or	1 lemon
corn oil, or combination	sea salt/pepper to taste
of both.	

Break egg into blender and process. While blender running, add oil in a thin stream until egg and oil thicken and do not separate. Squeeze in juice of lemon, add mustard, season to taste with salt/pepper and blend to combine.

Yields 1 1/2 cups.

✳

Basil Mayonnaise

1 egg, room temperature	1 tablespoon dried basil
1/2 to 3/4 cup olive oil	1 lemon
sea salt/pepper to taste	

Break egg into blender and process. With blender running, add oil in a thin stream until egg and oil thicken and do not separate. Squeeze in juice of lemon, add basil, season to taste and blend.

Yields 1 1/2 cups.

Curry Mayonnaise

1 egg, room temperature
1/2 - 3/4 cup oil
2 limes
1 shallot

1 tablespoon Dijon mustard
1 tablespoon curry powder
1 lemon

Break egg into blender and process. With blender running, add oil in a thin stream until egg and oil thicken and do not separate. Squeeze in juice of limes. Peel shallot and slice into blender and blend. Add mustard, curry powder and lemon and blend to combine.

Yields about 1 cup.

✳

Seafood Mayonnaise (Full of Life phase)
(for cold crab, prawns or lobster)

1 egg yolk, room temperature
1/2 cup virgin oil
1 tablespoon tomato catsup
sea salt/pepper to taste

1 tablespoon Dijon mustard
1 lemon
2 tablespoons white rum

Place egg yolk in blender and process. With blender running, add oil in a thin stream until egg and oil thicken and do not separate. Squeeze in juice of lemon, add mustard and blend. Add catsup and rum, and blend to combine. Pour dressing into a small bowl and season to taste with sea salt/pepper.

Yields 1 cup.

✳

Cashew Mayonnaise

1/2 cup cashews, rinsed
1 cup water
1/2 teaspoon onion powder

pinch garlic powder
1/2 teaspoon sea salt

Pour into saucepan and cook until thick, stirring constantly until creamy. Then add 2 tablespoons fresh lemon juice.

Tahini Mayonnaise (Second phase)

1 cup Tahini
1/4 cup fresh lemon juice
1 teaspoon sea salt

1/2 teaspoon garlic powder
1 teaspoon onion powder
1 cup water

Combine all the ingredients in blender.

✳

Tomato Cream Dressing

3 fresh tomatoes
2 tablespoon fresh lemon juice
1 teaspoon raw cashew nuts

1 tablespoon olive oil
1 teaspoon rice syrup

Combine all the ingredients in blender.

✳

Creamy Pasta Salad Dressing

1 cup plain yogurt, goats
1 teaspoon dill weed

1 tablespoon minced chives
1 tablespoon lemon juice

Mix ingredients together thoroughly and let stand in covered container in refrigerator for about half an hour before using.
Yields 1 cup.

✳

Easy Pasta Dressing

1/3 cup olive oil
juice from 1 lemon

1 clove garlic finely minced
1 bay leaf, slightly crumbled

Put oil in small jar. Add lemon juice and minced garlic. Crumble bay leaf to help release the flavor. Allow dressing to stand in covered container overnight or for several hours before using. Before dressing the salad, remove the bay leaf.
Yields approx. 2/3 cup dressing.

Easy Herb Dressing

1/3 cup vegetable oil
juice from 1 lemon
1 tablespoon sweet basil

1 tablespoon dill weed
1 tablespoon oregano

Mix all ingredients together several hours before dressing is to be used. Let stand in covered container to allow flavors to blend.
Yields about 2/3 cup dressing.

✳

Lemony Herb Dressing
(salad greens)

1 tablespoon rice syrup
1/2 teaspoon dry mustard
1/2 teaspoon dried basil leaves
1/3 cup lemon juice
1/4 teaspoon dried dill weed

1/2 teaspoon sea salt
1/4 teaspoon paprika
1/4 teaspoon garlic powder
3/4 cup salad oil

In a jar with a screw top, blend together all the dry ingredients. Add the lemon juice and oil. Screw on the jar lid and shake well. Chill. Shake well again just before serving.
Yields just over 1 cup.

✳

Zesty Salad Dressing

1/3 cup salad oil
1/4 cup lemon
1 clove garlic, finely minced

1/2 teaspoon ground cumin
1 teaspoon chili powder
 sea salt/pepper to taste

Mix all ingredients together in a small container (glass jar with lid). Shake covered container thoroughly to be sure ingredients are well mixed. Allow dressing to stand for 1/2 hour or more to be sure flavors are well mixed. Shake again, just before pouring.
Yields 1/2 cup.

Cucumber Dill Dressing
(salad greens/sprouts)

3 tablespoons mild oil
1 tablespoon lemon
1 teaspoon dill weed

1/2 cup parsley
1 teaspoon rice syrup
1 teaspoon celery seed

Blenderize above ingredients until creamy. Add a two-inch length of cucumber, chopped and blend until absolutely smooth.
Yields 3/4 cup.

✳

Parsley Dressing

2 scallions minced (1/4 cup)
1 cup low-fat goat cheese
1/2 cup tomato-vegetable juice

1 tablespoon lemon
1/3 cup chopped parsley

Combine all ingredients in blender and blend until smooth.

✳

Classic Garlic Dressing

1/2 cup lemon
2 tablespoons Dijon mustard
1/4 cup boiling water

1 teaspoon sea salt
1 tablespoon pressed fresh garlic
1/16 teaspoon white pepper

Whisk together the above ingredients...and whisk in, beating well:
1 cup vegetable oil & 1 cup olive oil
Set dressing aside to age before serving. Whisk again before serving.
Yields about 2 cups.

Remoulade Sauce
(chicken, hard cooked eggs, cheese)

1 cup mayonnaise
2 tablespoons chives, chopped
1 tablespoons parsley, chopped
3 tablespoons dill pickle, chopped

1/4 teaspoon horseradish
1/8 cup Dijon mustard
2 tablespoons scallions, chopped

Combine all ingredients and serve cold.
Servings, 4.

❋

Blue Cheese Dressing (Full of Life phase)

1/2 cup plain yogurt (goats)
1/2 cup sour cream
2 tablespoons blue cheese

dash milk (goats) if needed
1/2 clove garlic, finely minced

Place all ingredients in blender and blend on high speed until well mixed. Use only enough milk to thin dressing to desired consistency. Allow dressing to stand covered in refrigerator for several hours before using.
Yields 1 cup dressing.

❋

Cucumber Dill Salad Dressing

2 large cucumbers, washed and
     thinly sliced
1 teaspoon dill weed

2 tablespoons green onion,
     finely minced
1 cup plain yogurt (goats)

In a large bowl combine the above ingredients. Mix thoroughly until vegies are coated with dill weed and yogurt dressing. Cover and chill for at least 1 hour before eating.
Yields 2-3 servings.

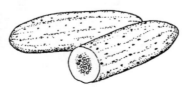

CHAPTER SEVEN

COOKING IN THE FAST LANE
QUICKIES

Hot Cream of Rice

1 cup brown rice
4 cups goats milk

1 teaspoon sea salt
rice or maple syrup

In a dry frying pan over medium heat, toast or "pop" the grains of rice for about 10 minutes, shaking the pan gently to prevent scorching. The grains should be slightly brown and smell nutty. Grind the grains in blender to the desired degree of coarseness. Bring goats milk and sea salt to a boil, then stir in ground grain. Cover the pan, lower the heat and simmer for 5 to 10 minutes. If you wish, sweeten to taste with rice syrup or maple syrup. Serve plain or with goats milk.
Serves 4.

Millet Mush

1 cup millet flour
4 cups water

corn oil
sea salt

Bring salted water to a oil, stir in millet, turn heat down and simmer over direct heat or transfer to top of double boiler, place over boiling water and cook, covered for 25 to 30 minutes, until millet is soft. Turn into oiled loaf pan and cool. Refrigerate overnight or for several hours. Remove from pan, slice loaf into 1/2-inch slices. Dust slices with flour and fry in a little oil until they are golden and crisp on both sides. Serve hot with maple syrup or honey.
Serves 4 to 6.

Nutty Hot Cereal

4 cups rolled oats
1 cup rolled barley
1 cup rolled rye

1 cup finely chopped nuts
   (filberts or almonds)

To cook a portion of cereal, bring 2 quarts of water to a boil. Add 1 part cereal mixture and stir. Reduce heat to a simmer and cook uncovered, stirring frequently, for about 20 minutes. Serve hot with milk goats milk and butter. Option: serve with honey.
   Makes 8 cups raw cereal.

※

Spanish Omelet

1/2 clove garlic
1 tablespoon butter
1 tablespoon olive oil
1 tablespoon onion, finely chopped
1 tablespoon watercress, chopped

1/2 cup tomatoes, peeled,
   seeded, diced and drained
1 tablespoon parsley, chopped
1 tablespoon green pepper,
   finely chopped

Cook the garlic in the olive oil and butter for 2 minutes, remove and discard. Add the onion, pepper, tomatoes, and parsley and sauté gently for 4 minutes. Add this mixture to a 3 egg French omelet before folding. Fold and serve garnished with chopped watercress.
   Serves 2.

※

Fresh Country Omelet

2 tablespoons butter
3 eggs well beaten

sea salt/pepper to taste
1/4 cup diced cooked

Melt butter in frying pan and add potatoes. Fry until potatoes are golden in color. Salt/pepper the eggs and pour into pan. Cook on low heat, lifting the edges to get the liquid eggs run to the bottom of the pan.
   Yields 2-3 servings.

Salsa Fria on Scrambled Eggs

1 small can tomato sauce	1 teaspoon lemon juice
1 clove garlic, finely chopped	1 tablespoon cilantro
1 small can chopped green chilies	dash sea salt

Mix all ingredients together in small bowl and refrigerate in covered container for several hours before serving. If you plan to serve this for breakfast prepare it the night before.
Makes a little over 1 cup salsa.

✳

East Indian Curry Eggs

2 eggs	dash sea salt
2 tablespoons butter	cayenne pepper
2 teaspoons curry powder	2 oz goats cheese, grated

Melt butter in saucepan. When hot stir in curry powder and fry lightly. Add goats cheese, sea salt, pepper, cayenne pepper. Lastly, stir in the slightly beaten eggs and cook until it reaches the consistency of scrambled eggs.

✳

Eggs/Tomatoes Provincial

2 tablespoons olive oil	4 tomatoes
1 clove garlic	2 eggs
2 tablespoons grated parmesan cheese	

Warm olive oil in a sauté pan over medium heat. Slice unpeeled tomatoes in pan. Peel garlic and slice into pan. Cook 5 minutes. Do not overcook tomatoes or they will lose their fresh flavor. Break eggs into pan on top of tomatoes, being careful to keep yolks intact. Cover eggs with grated cheese. Cover pan and cook for 2 or 3 minutes until eggs are set.

Monterey Jack Cheese Eggs

2 tablespoons olive oil
1 medium size red bell pepper
1 tomato
1 teaspoon dried basil
sea salt/pepper to taste

2 tablespoons cold water
1/4 cup grated Monterey
  Jack cheese
2 eggs

Warm olive oil in a sauté pan over medium heat. Thinly slice bell pepper into pan, discarding seeds and ribs and stir in basil. Simmer 2 minutes. Slice tomato into pan. Cover and cook for 2 minutes. Break eggs into a bowl, add water and whisk until well blended. Pour eggs in pan and add grated cheese and season to taste. Cover pan and cook for 2 minutes.

Poached Eggs Au Gratin

4 eggs
1 cup béchamel sauce

6 tablespoons grated
parmesan cheese

Poach the eggs and place them into a buttered shirring pan or into 2 individual ramekins. Sprinkle with Parmesan cheese, cover with béchamel sauce and top with more cheese. Bake in a preheated 350 degree oven until top is brown (about 4 minutes).
Serves 2.

Béchamel Sauce
(Basic White Sauce)

4 tablespoons butter
1/2 teaspoon sea salt
pepper/pinch

4 tablespoons rice flour
2 cups hot goats milk

Put all the ingredients into an electric blender and blend for 1/2 a minute at full speed. Pour into saucepan and cook over low heat for 10 minutes, stirring constantly. To make a thicker sauce, use 6 tablespoons rice flour instead of 4.
Yields 2 cups.

<u>VARIATIONS:</u>

CURRY SAUCE: Add before cooking, 1 teaspoon curry powder.

Potato Pancakes

1 large red potato	2 tablespoons chopped chives
1 slice onion	1 tablespoon olive oil
1 egg	1/4 baking powder
1/4 cup goats milk	black pepper to taste
1/4 cup rice flour	

Scrub the potato well and slice it and the onion into blender or food processor. Add egg and goats milk and puree. Add rice flour and baking powder. Blend until lumps disappear, about 5 seconds. Warm olive oil in a sauté pan over medium heat. When hot, pour tablespoons of batter into pan. Cook about 2 minutes on each side. Turn when golden brown. Season to taste with pepper, sprinkle chives over pancakes and serve at once.

Yields 8 pancakes.

Soup Croutons

1/2 loaf French or Italian sourdough bread	1/4 cup grated parmesan cheese or to taste
1 garlic clove, peeled	2 tablespoons olive oil

Rub the crust of the bread all over with the garlic clove. Cut the bread into 1/8 inch thick slices and arrange the slices on a baking sheet. Sprinkle with the oil and the cheese. Broil until golden on both sides, then cut into 1-inch squares.

Yields about 12 croutons.

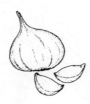

Garlic Soup
(Healthy soup for colds and flu)

1 large head fresh garlic
2 quarts chicken broth
1 quart water
3 cups diced potatoes
2 cloves

4 sprigs parsley
3 tablespoons olive oil
pinch thyme
pinch sage

Separate the garlic cloves and peel by laying on a cutting board and slapping hard with the flat side of a large-bladed knife or cleaver. The skin will fall away. Combine the garlic, water, cloves, thyme, sage and olive oil; simmer in the chicken broth, covered, 30 minutes. Add the potatoes and simmer another 20 minutes. Put through the blender, reheat and serve.

VARIATION:
Leave out the potatoes but simmer the additional time and pour over a thick slice of toasted French bread in each bowl.

✳

Rosemary Soup

1 tablespoon dried rosemary
  (or 2 tablespoons fresh)
1 cup sorrel
1 cup watercress
1 head lettuce

3 tablespoons butter
1 egg yolk
sea salt/pepper to taste
1/2 cup cream
1 1/2 quarts chicken stock
  (or half water)

Cook the rosemary, sorrel, watercress and lettuce in butter for about 5 minutes, all shredded or cut fine. Add stock and simmer a half hour. Mix the egg yolk with the cream and stir into the mixture just before taking off the fire. Add sea salt/pepper to taste.

Cold Avocado Soup

1 cup chicken broth
1 small ripe avocado
1 teaspoon dried oregano
sea salt/pepper to taste

1/2 cup sour cream
1 lemon
2 lemon slices (optional)

Place broth in a saucepan over high heat. Peel avocado and slice into blender or food processor. Add oregano and squeeze in juice of lemon. Add sour cream and blend all ingredients together well. Place puree in a bowl, stir in broth and season to taste with sea salt/pepper. Serve cold or at room temperature. (Optional: garnish with thin slices of lemon).

✳

Watercress Soup

2 bunches watercress
1 quart chicken stock
  (or half water)
1 sprig thyme
1 onion, minced
1 bay leaf

3 tablespoons butter
sea salt/pepper to taste
paprika
1 egg yolk
1/4 cup cream

Wash the watercress carefully, then chop fine. Peel and dice the potatoes. Melt the butter in a deep skilled; add the watercress and the onion, bay leaf and thyme. When the watercress is limp, add the potatoes and cover with the chicken stock. Simmer with the egg yolk stirred into the cream. Serve at once, garnished with chopped watercress and parsley.

✳

Okra Creole

2 dozen okras
2 medium fresh tomatoes
  (or 1/2 cup canned tomatoes)
1 onion, minced
1/2 green pepper, minced

1 tablespoon butter
1/teaspoon minced parsley
1/2 clove garlic, minced
sea salt/pepper to taste
cayenne

Wash okras and cut off ends. Put in saucepan with butter, onion, garlic and green pepper and cook about 10 minutes. Add tomatoes (cut up into small pieces and the juice). Add salt/pepper to taste, parsley, cayenne, and the okras and simmer 20 minutes.

*

Carrot Puree Soup

3 cups chicken broth	1 shallot
4 medium size carrots	1 teaspoon dried thyme
black pepper to taste	

Place broth in a saucepan over high heat. Coarsely chop carrots and place in broth. Peel shallot and slice into broth and add thyme. Boil rapidly over high heat for 8 minutes. Place vegetables and broth in blender (or food processor) and puree. Season to taste with pepper.
   Yields 3 cups.

*

Gazpacho Soup

1 cup alfalfa sprouts	1 stalk celery, chopped
4 cups tomato juice	1/2 cucumber, chopped
2 medium-size tomatoes,	1 green onion, chopped
skinned and chopped	1 1-inch slice green pepper
	chopped

Combine all ingredients in blender and process until completely liquefied. Chill 1 hour.
   Yields 6 cups.

*

Yellow Squash Puree Soup
(15 minutes)

3 cups chicken broth	1 teaspoon curry powder
4 yellow squash or yellow	black pepper to taste
zucchini	2 scallions
1/2 cup heavy cream	

Pour broth into a saucepan and place over high heat. Coarsely chop squash and scallions and place in broth. Boil rapidly over high heat for 5 minutes. Place squash and broth in blender (or food processor) and puree. Add cream and curry and blend. Season to taste with pepper.

Yields 4 cups.

Bohemian Veggie Soup

2 tablespoons barley	1 medium potato
boiled 1 hour in	4 stalks celery
2 quarts of water	3 small carrots
2 small onions	1 turnip
2 tablespoons rice flour	sea salt/pepper to taste
3 tablespoons butter	

Grate all vegetables in blender and put into the barley water, add onions and cook slowly. Add sea salt/pepper to taste. Then thicken with 2 tablespoons rice flour, slightly burnt and cooked with 3 tablespoons of melted butter and add to barley water. Boil up and serve.

✳

Apricot Soup

4 cups pitted fresh apricots	6 tablespoons rice syrup
2 cups water	1/4 cup cornstarch
1/2 teaspoon almond extract	1/4 cup water
(optional)	

Combine apricots and water in a saucepan and bring to a boil. Turn heat down and simmer for 5 minutes or until apricots are tender but still firm. Lift out about 1 cup apricots and set aside. Puree remaining apricots and (1 1/4 cup) water in blender. Return puree to saucepan and heat. Add rice syrup. Dissolve cornstarch in water and stir into puree when it is boiling. Continue to cook, stirring, for about 1 minute, until soup is thickened and clear. Remove from heat, add almond extract, if desired, and cool. Cut reserved apricots into quarters and add to soup. Chill completely before serving.

Yields 4 servings.

Chilled Beet Soup

2 medium beets, cooked	1 quart boiling water
1 teaspoon sea salt	1 egg, beaten
2 teaspoons rice syrup	1/3 cup yogurt, goats
2 teaspoons lemon juice	

Remove beet skins. Chop beets fine and cook in boiling salted water until beets are soft. Add egg, rice syrup and lemon juice and mix. Chill. Top with yogurt (goats).
Serves 2.

❋

Cold Whey Soup with Potatoes/Zucchini

1 cup chopped celery including leaves	1/2 teaspoon dill
1 cup chopped onion	1/2 teaspoon basil
2 cups diced potatoes	1/2 teaspoon sea salt
2 cups diced zucchini	1/8 teaspoon pepper
4 cups whey or soup stock	2 tablespoons chopped parsley

In a large sauce pan, combine celery, onion, potatoes and zucchini. Cover with water, add seasonings and simmer for about 15 minutes or until vegetables are just tender. Add whey or stock, bring to a boil and simmer for 2 or 3 minutes longer. Cool and then chill in refrigerator for at least an hour. Serve topped with chopped parsley.
Yields approx. 6 cups.

❋

Russian Soup

1/2 cup barley	1/2 teaspoon dried mint
2 cups chicken stock	sea salt to taste
1 small onion, minced	2 eggs beaten
1 tablespoon butter	1 cup yogurt, goats
1 tablespoon rye or whole wheat flour	1/4 teaspoon ground coriander
fresh mint, chopped	fresh parsley, chopped
2 tablespoons fresh lemon juice	1/4 teaspoon lemon juice
dill	

Cook barley according to preferred method. Sauté onion in butter. Heat chicken stock to boiling and stir onion and cooked barley with any remaining liquid into stock. Add herbs and sea salt. Blend flour into eggs, then carefully stir in yogurt. Add a little of the hot soup to the egg and yogurt mixture, gradually stirring it in to avoid "scrambling" the eggs, then our this back into the hot soup. Stir in lemon juice. Keep hot but do not boil. Add fresh parsley and mint just before serving.

Serves 6 to 8.

Gourmet Lentil

2 tablespoons olive oil
1 cup finely chopped onions
2 teaspoons garlic, finely chopped
1/2 cup lentils
1/2 cup uncooked rice
6 cups fresh chicken broth

1 bay leaf
1 teaspoon dried thyme or
2 sprigs of fresh thyme
2 tablespoons parsley, finely chopped
sea salt/pepper to taste
2 cups water

Heat the olive oil in a deep sauce pan. Add the onions and garlic. Cook briefly, stirring until wilted. Do not brown. Add the lentils, rice, broth, water, bay leaf, thyme, sea salt and pepper. Simmer 30 minutes. Scoop out 1 cup of the lentils, rice and broth and set aside. Remove and discard bay leaf. Put the remaining soup through a food processor or food mill and process until fine. This may have to be done in two or more operations. Return the soup to the pan and add the reserved cup. Add the cream and bring to a simmer. Adjust the seasonings. Sprinkle with parsley (or chervil). Serve piping hot with croutons.

Serves 4.

Leek and Potato Soup

2 large leeks
1 Lb medium potatoes, like yellow gold or Washington
4 tablespoons butter
1 cup finely chopped onion

3 cups fresh chicken stock
2 cups water
1 bay leaf
sea salt/pepper to taste

Leeks have a great deal of sand between the leaves and must be carefully cleaned. To do this, trim off the root end and cut off and discard the long green stems. Split the leeks lengthwise from the stem end, then turn and split them one more time. Rinse well. Separate the leaves under cold running water, then chop into 1/4 inch pieces. Peel the potatoes and cut them into 1/4 inch cubes (about 2 cups). Melt 2 tablespoons of the butter in a sauce pan; add the onions and the chopped leeks. Cook over medium heat, stirring, until wilted. Do not brown. Add the chicken broth, water, bay leaf, add the remaining butter and stir. Adjust the seasonings and serve piping hot with croutons. Yields 4 to 6 servings. Note: For a richer version, stir in 1/2 cup drained plain yogurt (goats) just before serving.

✳

Oatmeal Soup

1/2 cup oatmeal	3/4 cup chopped tomato
1/2 small onion, finely chopped	1 large clove garlic, minced
1 tablespoon melted butter	4 cups any soup stock
1/4 teaspoon sea salt	2 teaspoons tamari soy sauce
2 tablespoons soy grits	

In an iron skillet or heavy-bottom sauce pan, roast oatmeal over medium-high heat, stirring constantly to keep it from burning, until it is light brown. Remove oatmeal from pan and set aside. Sauté onion and garlic in oil or butter until tender. Combine with tomato, stock, soy grits and tasted oatmeal and cook over low heat approximately 5 minutes. Season with tamari soy sauce, sea salt and serve.

Yields approximately 4 cups.

✳

Smoked Salmon Open-Face Sandwich

Cover toasted, buttered rye bread with smoked salmon and hot scrambled eggs.

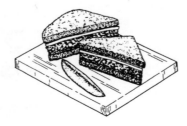

Quick Chili Sandwiches

1 tablespoon olive oil
1 tablespoon chopped onion
1 tablespoon chopped onion
dash tabasco or salsa

1/2 Lb ground turkey
1 teaspoon chili powder
1/4 teaspoon cumin seed

Mix all the ingredients and sauté in a hot skilled for 10 minutes. Serve between slices of heated rolls.
Serves 2.

✳

Chicken and Celery Sandwich Filling

1 cup minced cooked chicken
  or turkey
1 tablespoon minced green

4 tablespoons mayonnaise
1/4 teaspoon sea salt
dash pepper
1 cup minced celery

Mix all ingredients together thoroughly.
Yields approx. 2 cups.

✳

Chicken and Cucumber Sandwich Filling

2 cups diced cooked chicken
1/2 cup diced cucumbers

1/2 cup chopped celery
3/4 cups mayonnaise

Mix all ingredients thoroughly.
Yields 2 cups.

✳

Chicken and Almond Sandwiches

1 cup cooked chicken meat,
  ground (or turkey)
1/2 cup minced celery
1/4 cup ground almonds

1/4 cup mayonnaise
8 slices toast
4 lettuce leaves

Mix chicken (or turkey), celery and almonds. Moisten with mayonnaise or salad dressing. Spread on buttered toast, cover with lettuce and a second slice of toast.

Makes 4 sandwiches

*

Crab-meat Sandwich Filling

1 1/2 cups cooked crab meat
3/4 cup diced celery
1 tablespoon diced green pepper

mayonnaise
1/4 teaspoon sea salt

Shred crab meat and discard all tough spines. Mix crab meat, celery, green pepper, salt and add enough mayonnaise to moisten.

Serves 4.

*

Sloppy Joe Turkey Sandwiches

1/2 cup chopped onion
1/2 cup chopped green pepper
2 tablespoons oil
1 1/2 Lbs ground turkey
  or chicken

1 tomato, peeled, squeezed,
  and chopped
1 teaspoon paprika
1 teaspoon sea salt

Using a heavy skillet, sauté the onion and green pepper in the oil until slightly brown. Add the remaining ingredients including the meat (loose). Cook over low heat 15 minutes, stirring often.

Serves 4.

Muffin Pizza

2 muffins, split and toasted
4 slices mozzarella cheese

pesto pasta sauce
1/2 teaspoon oregano

Spread the muffin halves generously with sauce, cover with slices of cheese and sprinkle with oregano. Slide under the broiler and cook until the cheese melts.

Serves 2.

Salmon and Cucumber Sandwich Filling

1 cup flaked cooked salmon   1/2 cup mayonnaise
1/4 cup chopped cucumber

Mix the above ingredients thoroughly.

✳

Salmon and Nut Sandwich Filling

1 cup flaked cooked salmon   1/2 cup mayonnaise
3 tablespoons minced celery   3 tablespoons chopped nut

Mix the above ingredients thoroughly.

✳

Lamb Sandwich

1 1/2 cups chopped cooked lamb   1/2 tablespoon minced onion
1 teaspoon minced mint leaves   1 tablespoon lemon juice
                                                             sea salt/pepper to taste

Mix the above ingredients thoroughly.
  Serves 2.

✳

Cheese Soufflé Sandwiches

8 slices bread   1 cup grated cheddar cheese
4 eggs, separated   (goats)
dash pepper   dash paprika
1/8 teaspoon sea salt

Remove crusts and toast bread on 1 side. Combine sea salt, pepper, paprika and egg yolks and beat until light. Fold yolks and grated cheddar cheese (goats) into stiffly beaten egg whites.   Heap onto untoasted side of bread and bake at 350 degrees for about 15 minutes or until puffy and brown.

Serves 8.

Fried Egg Sandwiches

1 small onion, minced	1/8 teaspoon sea salt
1 small green pepper, minced	dash pepper
2 tablespoons butter	4 slices toast
1 cup cooked tomatoes	4 fried eggs
grated goats cheese	

Cook onion and green pepper in butter until tender. Add tomatoes, sea salt and pepper and cook until reduced one-half. Spread sauce on each slice and cover egg with grated goats cheese. Melt cheese under broiler. Serve hot.

Makes 4 sandwiches.

Waffle Sandwich

Split thin baking powder biscuits, butter and top with a slice of tomato and a slice of cheese. Melt cheese under broiler.

✳

Sliced Turkey Sandwiches

8 slices bread	sea salt/pepper to taste
slices turkey or chicken	mayonnaise
lettuce	

Spread bread with butter. Cover 4 slices with turkey, sprinkle with sea salt and pepper, spread with mayonnaise and top with lettuce and remaining slices of bread.   Cut diagonally into quarters.

Serves 4.

Curry Burgers

1 Lb ground turkey meat
1 egg
1/2 cup crushed pineapple
1 banana, finely chopped
chutney

1 teaspoon Worcestershire
    sauce
1 teaspoon curry powder
4-6 buns

Mix meat and egg thoroughly.   Add pineapple and banana.   Mix well. Add Worcestershire sauce and curry powder. Mix seasonings in thoroughly. Form 4-6 patties. Bake patties in oven until done to your taste. Spread bun halves with chutney. Add the cooked patties and serve.

Serves about 4-6.

✳

Taco Burgers

1 Lb ground turkey meat
1 egg
1 tablespoon chopped onion
1/2 teaspoon chili powder, or
   to your taste

1/2 cup chili salsa
shredded lettuce
4-6 slices tomato
4-6 slices cheddar cheese (goats)
4-6 wheat buns

Mix meat, egg, onion, chili powder and chili salsa. Form meat mixture into patties and cook. Open buns and on the bottom halves layer shredded lettuce, the tomato slices and the cheese slices. Add the cooked patties and the bun tops.

Serves 4-6.

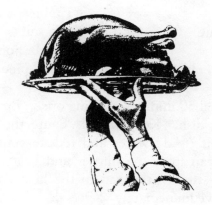

Salad Burgers

1 Lb ground turkey meat
1 egg
1/4 cup grated carrot
1/4 cup thin sliced celery
1/4 cup grated zucchini
4-6 slices tomato
4-6 buns

1 tablespoon finely chopped
   green pepper
1 teaspoon chopped onion
shredded lettuce or fresh
spinach leaves
special sauce (see below)

Mix meat, egg, carrot, celery, zucchini, green pepper and onion together., Form mixture into meat patties (about 4-6). Bake patties at 350 degrees for about 20 minutes or until cooked to your taste. While meat is cooking mix the Special Sauce.

Special Sauce
(for Salad Burgers)

1/2 cup mayonnaise

1 teaspoon mustard

Mix sauce ingredients together in a small dish. Open the buns and spread sauce on bottom halves. Add the lettuce or spinach leaves and tomato slices. Add cooked meat patties. Top them with the top halves of the buns.
Serves 4-6.

Salmon Steaks with Butter Sauce

2 Lbs salmon steaks
2 tablespoons margarine
4 shallots, minced
1 1/2 sticks margarine, chilled and cut into small pieces

1 tablespoon olive oil
 sea salt
4 tablespoons water

Marinate the fish in the olive oil 30 minutes, turning once. Broil 7 minutes on each side, and arrange on a hot serving dish. Keep warm. Sauté the shallots very gently in 1 tablespoon margarine until soft. Add water and reduce gently until 2 tablespoons of liquid remain. Remove the pan from the burner and beat in 2 pieces of the chilled margarine with a wire whisk. Return the pan to the heat and beat in the rest of the margarine pieces by piece. Serve immediately. *Serves 4.*

Millet Stuffed Peppers

1/2 cup millet
1 medium-size onion, minced
1/2 Lb ground beef (organic)
2 tablespoons chopped parsley
1 teaspoon oregano

4 green peppers, halved
 cored and seeded
1 tablespoon corn oil
2 tablespoons wheat germ
1 tablespoon parmesan
 cheese

Cook millet according to preferred method. Steam peppers for 5 minutes. Sauté onion and beef in oil for about 5 minutes, stirring to brown meat evenly. Preheat oven to 350 degrees. Combine millet with meat mixture, add seasonings and stuff into pepper halves. Top with wheat germ and parmesan cheese and bake in preheated oven for 20 minutes. Serve with your favorite Tomato Sauce.
Serves 4.

✳

Broiled Fillets of Sole

6 sole fillets, large/firm
2 tablespoons parsley, chopped
4 tablespoons olive oil
1 teaspoon basil

1 clove garlic, crushed
1 teaspoon sea salt
3 shallots, minced

Sauté the shallots and garlic in the olive oil. Add the basil and sea salt. Simmer about 5 minutes. Brush the fillets with olive oil and place on the broiler rack. Broil 5 minutes, turn, pour the sauce over them and continue broiling another 4 or 5 minutes until the fish is done.
Serves 6.

✳

Broiled Sole with Herbs

2 tablespoons chopped chives
6 sole fillets
1 tsp. tarragon

1 stick butter
1 1/2 tsp. sea salt

Place the fillets on an oiled broiling rack and spread with the mixture of the other ingredients. Broil for approximately 4 minutes on each side.

Serves 6.

Scallops Amandine

1 Lb scallops
1/3 cup butter
1/2 cup slivered toasted almonds

rice flour
2tablespoons chopped parsley

Cut the scallops into bite-size pieces if large; dust with flour and brown in half the butter until crisp and golden. Arrange on a heated serving dish. Melt the remaining butter, add the almonds and parsley, and pour this over the scallops.

Serves 4.

*

Lobster Dream

2 cups lobster meat
4 tablespoons rice flour
1 cup cream
paprika

1 teaspoon tarragon,
sea salt/pepper to taste
4 tablespoons butter
3 hard-boiled eggs

Press egg whites through a coarse sieve. Mash egg yolks and moisten with a little cream. Rub flour into butter until smooth; melt in sauce pan, add lobster, egg yolks and whites, and the rest of the cream. Stir until well heated; add salt/pepper and dust thickly with paprika, adding minced tarragon at the last.

Serves 4.

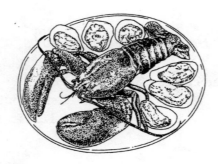

Broiled Fish

2 Lbs fish filleted: halibut	sea salt/pepper to taste
(or salmon, whitefish)	rice flour (or cornmeal)
light olive oil	

Preheat broiler. Dip fish in oil. Season and sprinkle lightly with rice flour or cornmeal. Place under broiler until done and brown on one side. Turn over and complete cooking. Serve with melted butter and lemon quarters.

Serves 4.

✳

Frog Legs Provincial

8 frog legs	4 cloves garlic, crushed
2 tablespoons finely chopped	5 tablespoons margarine
parsley	2 tablespoons finely
2 tablespoons finely chopped	chopped tarragon
chives	sea salt
rice flour	

Wash the frog legs, dry and dust lightly with salted rice flour. Melt the margarine and add the garlic. Cook 1 minute then add the frog legs and sauté until golden brown on both sides. Add the parsley, chives and tarragon, taste for seasoning and cook for 1 minute more, or until a fork tests shows they are done.

Serves 2.

✳

Chicken Paprika

1 3-Lb frying chicken	1 medium onion, chopped
(cut into 8 pieces)	1 tablespoon paprika
3 tablespoons butter	pinch curry powder
3 tablespoons rice flour	1 quart chicken stock
1/2 cup sour cream at room	1 teaspoon sea salt
temperature	1/8 teaspoon pepper

Season chicken. Dredge in rice flour and fry in butter until golden brown. Add onions and cook with chicken for about 10 to 15 minutes. Add seasonings and chicken stock and cook an additional 45 minutes or until cooked. Remove chicken to a warm platter. Bring gravy to a boil and add sour cream (or non-dairy sour cream substitute). Mix well and pour over chicken.

Yields approx. 4 servings.

✻

Lamb Kebabs

4 tablespoons olive oil
1/2 Lb lamb cubes cut from leg
1 lemon
sea salt/pepper to taste

1 small eggplant
10 small cherry tomatoes
1 teaspoon dried oregano

Preheat broiler. Pour olive oil into a bowl and squeeze in juice of lemon. Add oregano and stir. Cut unpeeled eggplant into cubes and toss in sauce mixture. Thread cubes of lamb on skewers, alternating with tomatoes and eggplant. Place in a baking dish. Pour remaining sauce over meat and vegetables and place under broiler about 3 inches from source of heat. Broil 6 minutes, turning skewers as lamb cooks. Season to taste and serve at once.

Serves 4.

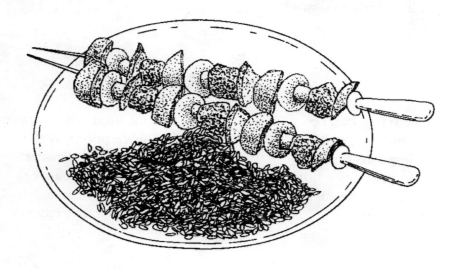

Creamy Crab on Rice

2 tablespoons olive oil
2 tablespoons butter
dash paprika
1 clove garlic, finely minced
2 cups cooked, shredded crab meat

1/4 cup rice flour
1/4 cup goats milk
1/2 cup yogurt, goats

In large skillet, heat olive oil and butter, until butter is melted. Add garlic and sauté over medium low heat. Add rice flour, stirring well. Add goats milk, slowly, stirring well to keep sauce from getting lumpy. Add yogurt and stir well. Add cooked crab and simmer, covered, for about 5 minutes or until mixture is thoroughly heated. Serve over hot brown rice and garnish with a dash of paprika.

Serves about 4.

Curried Crab with Rice

2 cups cooked crab meat, fresh,
   canned or frozen
2 tablespoons unsalted butter
1/2 cup heavy cream or canned
   coconut milk

2 limes
2 teaspoons curry
1/4 tsp. cayenne pepper

Finely chopped scallions. Melt butter in a sauté pan over medium heat, stir scallions into pan, and sauté until soft, about 2 minutes. Stir in curry powder and cook 1 minute. Add crab meat and cayenne pepper and squeeze in juice of limes. Sauté 1 minute. Pour in cream (or coconut milk) and simmer over high heat for 2 minutes. Serve at once on a bed of rice.

Serves 4.

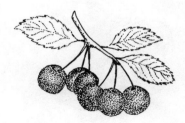

Red Snapper with Orange Sauce

2 tablespoons olive oil	sea salt/pepper to taste
2 red snapper fillets,	1 orange
(3/4 Lb) boned/skinned	paprika
2 bay leaves	

Warm oil in a sauté pan over medium heat, add bay leaves, and place fish in pan. Cut thin slices from unpeeled orange and place 1 on each slice of fish. Squeeze juice of orange over fish. Cover pan and cook for 6 minutes until fish is white and opaque and flakes easily when tested with a fork. Season to taste, dust with paprika and serve at once.

Serves 2.

✳

Lamb Patties with Red/Yellow Peppers

1/2 Lb ground lamb	2 teaspoons dried thyme
1 lemon	1 small red bell pepper
1 egg	1 small yellow bell pepper
1 small yellow onion	sea salt/pepper to taste

Place lamb in blender or food processor. Add juice of 1/2 lemon. Peel onion and slice into blender, add egg and blend well. Warm oil in a sauté pan over medium heat, add thyme and stir for a few seconds. Cut peppers into strips, discarding seeds and ribs. Place peppers in pan and stir until peppers become soft. With a tablespoon shape small patties of lamb mixture and flatten them with the back of the spoon. Place lamb patties in hot oil with red/yellow bell peppers and cook for 2 or 3 minutes on each side, until golden and crusty. Season to taste with sea salt/black pepper. Serve with rice and garnish with remaining 1/2 lemon.

Serves 2.

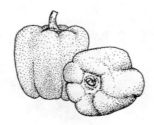

Turkey Pie with Sweet Potato Crust

3 cups diced cooked turkey
6 cooked small white onions
1 tablespoon chopped parsley
1 teaspoon sea salt
1/2 cup yogurt, goats

1 cup diced cooked carrots
1/2 cup goats milk
1 cup turkey stock
1/2 teaspoon pepper

Arrange turkey, carrots, onions and parsley in layers in casserole. Combine goats milk, yogurt and turkey stock and add slowly to flour blending well. Cook until thickened, stirring constantly. Season and pour over turkey and vegetables in casserole. Cover with Sweet Potato Crust recipe (see below). Bake in moderate oven at 350 degrees about 40 minutes.

Serves 6 to 8.

✳

Sweet Potato Crust

1 cup sifted rice flour
1 egg, well beaten
1 teaspoon baking powder

1 cup cold mashed sweet potato
1/2 teaspoon sea salt
1 Tbs. corn oil

Sift rice flour with baking powder and salt. Work in mashed potato, corn oil and egg. Roll 1/4 inch thick and cover turkey pie.

✳

Oat Pilaf
(serve with broiled chicken)

2 cups regular oatmeal
2 eggs
1 teaspoon poultry seasoning
sea salt/pepper to taste

1/2 teaspoon rubbed sage
2 Tbs corn oil
1 cup defatted chicken broth

In a medium size bowl combine the oats and the eggs. Just stir the egg into the oats and mix well until oats are covered with egg. Let this stand for 5 minutes. In a large skillet, heat the butter and oil until it is hot enough to sauté. Add the oats and toast in the oil, stirring frequently. Toast the oats until they are golden brown and in small clumps like ground beef. Add the garlic, onion, celery, poultry seasoning and salt/pepper. Cook gently until vegetables are beginning to soften, about 3 minutes. Add the chicken broth and cook until all liquid is absorbed, about 5 minutes. Serve hot.

Serves 6.

*

Cumin Chicken (or Turkey)

Mix:

1 small carton plain yogurt, goats	3 cloves garlic, crushed
1 teaspoon ground turmeric	1 medium onion, chopped
1/2 teaspoon ground cumin	1 teaspoon sea salt
1/2 teaspoon ground coriander	1 inch piece ginger root, finely diced
1 large lemon, rind and juice, finely grated and squeezed	1/2 teaspoon finely chopped green chilies

Place in oven-proof dish:

4 large chicken or turkey pieces

Pour yogurt mixture over and marinate for 1 to 2 hours, turning from time to time. Cover with foil and bake 45 to 60 minutes at 375 degrees, until chicken (turkey) is tender. Serve with brown rice.

Serves 4.

*

Broiled Tuna

2 slices tuna (3/4 Lb)	1 teaspoon powdered ginger
3 tablespoons olive oil	1 lemon
1/4 cup dry vermouth	

Preheat broiler. Place fish on baking sheet. Pour oil into a small bowl and squeeze in juice of lemon. Add ginger and vermouth. Stir to combine well. Coat both sides of fish with sauce. Place sheet on oven rack 3 to 4 inches from the source of heat. Broil fish 3 to 4 minutes on each side, until golden, and baste with sauce while cooking. When done, fish will flake when tested with a fork. Serve with special Tuna Cucumber Sauce listed below.

Serves 2.

Tuna Cucumber Sauce

1 cucumber	1 teaspoon Dijon mustard
1/2 cup olive oil	cayenne pepper
1/2 teaspoon dried thyme	1 lemon

With a sharp knife peel cucumber, leaving a few stripes of peel, and finely chop. Pour oil into a small bowl. Add thyme, mustard and a pinch of cayenne pepper. Squeeze in juice of lemon and stir in chopped cucumber.

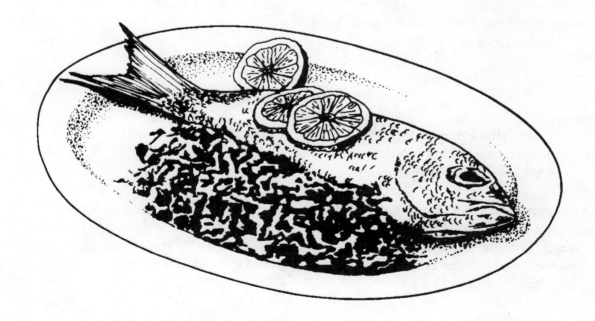

CHAPTER EIGHT

Biscuits - Muffins - Breads - Popovers - Crackers

BISCUITS

Rice Flour Biscuits
(preheat oven 400 degrees)

2 cups brown rice flour
1 teaspoon sea salt
1 cup goats milk
1 tablespoon corn oil

2 tablespoons rice syrup
3 egg yolks, slightly
 beaten

Combine all ingredients except egg whites. Mix thoroughly and beat with whisk until light (about 2 minutes). Fold in egg whites. Pour into oiled muffin tins and bake in preheated oven for 20 minutes, or until done.

Makes 12 muffins.

✳

Baking Powder Biscuits

2 cups sifted rice flour
3 teaspoons baking powder
4 tablespoons cold shortening

1/2 teaspoon sea salt
3/4 cup goats milk

Sift dry ingredients together and cut in shortening. Add goats milk to make a soft dough. Place on a floured board and knead lightly a few seconds, using as little flour as possible on board. Roll out 1/2 inch thick and cut with floured biscuit cutter. Place on greased baking sheet and bake in very hot oven at 450 degrees for about 12 minutes.

Makes 14 (2 inch) biscuits.

Sweet Potato Biscuits

1 1/2 cups sifted rice flour
2 tablespoons baking powder
1 1/2 cups mashed sweet potatoes

1/2 cup cold shortening
1 cup goats milk
3/4 teaspoons sea salt

Sift flour, baking powder and salt together. Cut in shortening. Combine goats milk and sweet potatoes. Add to first mixture and stir quickly. Knead lightly, using as little flour as possible on board. Roll out to 1/2 inch thickness, cut with floured cutter. Place on greased baking sheet and bake in hot oven at 425 degrees for 12 to 15 minutes.
Makes 25 biscuits.

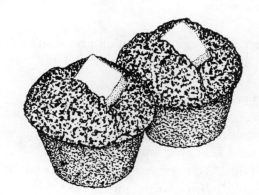

MUFFINS

Barley Muffins

1 cup barley flour
2 teaspoons baking powder
1 teaspoon soda
2 teaspoons cinnamon
1/4 cup safflower or corn oil

1 tablespoon orange rind
1/2 cup orange juice
1/2 cup mild honey
1 egg white, beaten

Sift together dry ingredients and orange rind. Combine liquid ingredients and beat with mixer or by hand. Stir liquid ingredients into dry until all is moistened well. Fold in beaten egg white. Fill prepared muffin pans full. Bake at 350 degrees for 20-25 minutes.
Makes 12.

✳

Basic Muffins

2 cups sifted, rice flour	1 egg, beaten
4 teaspoons baking powder	1 cup goats milk
1/2 teaspoon sea salt	1/4 cup rice syrup
1/4 cup melted shortening	

Sift dry ingredients together. Mix egg, shortening and goats milk mixtures, stirring just enough to dampen flour. Fill greased muffin pans 2/3 full. Bake in hot oven at 400 degrees for 25 minutes.
Makes 12 to 15 muffins.

Variations:

Blueberry - add 1 cup blueberries to dry ingredients.
Nut   - add 1/3 cup chopped nuts.
Cheese - add 1/2 cup grated goats cheese and 1/8 teaspoon paprika.
Pineapple - add 1 cup crushed pineapple to dry ingredients.

✳

Sunflower Seed Muffins (second phase)
(preheat oven 375 degrees)

3/4 cup sunflower seed meal (ground to a meal in blender)	1/4 teaspoon sea salt
	2 tablespoons rice syrup
3/4 cup whole wheat flour	3/4 cup goats milk
2 egg yolks	1 tablespoon corn oil
2 egg whites, well beaten	3/4 cup raisins

In a bowl combine flour, unflower seed meal and sea salt. In another bowl, beat egg yokes, then add oil, rice syrup, goats milk and raisins. Combine wet and dry mixtures. Fold in beaten egg whites. Bake in oiled muffin tins in preheated oven for 25 minutes.
Yields 12 muffins.

Basic Barley Flour Muffins

1 1/2 cups barley flour	1 teaspoon rice syrup
1 tablespoon baking powder	1 tablespoon honey
1 cup goats milk	3 tablespoons melted butter
1 egg	

Combine dry ingredients well. Beat the liquid ingredients together with a fork and combine with the dry ingredients using a minimum of strokes. Fill greased muffin pans 2/3 full and bake at 350 degrees for 15-20 minutes.

Carrot Muffins

Combine dry ingredients:

> 2 cups whole-wheat pastry flour
> 1/4 cup wheat germ
> 1 tablespoon (no aluminum) baking powder
> 1/2 teaspoon powdered nutmeg
> 1/2 teaspoon powdered ginger
> 3/4 teaspoon cinnamon

Separately Combine:

> 1/2 cup goats milk
> 1/2 cup light vegetable oil
> 1/2 cup honey
> 3 eggs
> 3/4 teaspoon vanilla extract

Stir liquid into dry ingredients. Mix, but do not beat.
FOLD IN: 1 1/2 cups carrots, finely grated
                1/2 cup currants
Spoon batter into buttered muffin cups or paper-lined cups. Fill cups almost to top, and garnish each muffin with a walnut. Bake 15 minutes at 400 degrees, preheated.

> *Yields 16 large muffins, or 12 large and 10 mini-muffins. NOTE: The mini-muffins only bake for 8 minutes.*

Cereal Flake Pecan Muffins

1 cup rice flour, sifted
1/4 teaspoon sea salt
2 1/2 teaspoons baking powder
3 tablespoons melted shortening

1/2 cup corn flakes
2/3 cup goats milk
1 egg, beaten
2 tablespoons rice syrup

Sift rice flour, baking powder and sea salt. Crush corn flakes and add; then add pecans. Combine egg, goats milk, rice syrup and shortening; add to flour mixture, stirring only enough to dampen all flour. Bake in greased muffin pans in hot oven at 425 degrees for 25 minutes.

Makes 10 muffins.

✳

Good Morning Muffins

2 cups whole-wheat flour
2 teaspoons baking soda
2 teaspoons cinnamon
1/2 cup bran
1/2 cup raw, chopped mixed nuts
1/2 cup raw sunflower seeds
1 cup cold-pressed vegetable oil

2 apples, cored/grated
2 teaspoons vanilla
3 large eggs
1/2 teaspoon sea salt
2 cups grated carrots
3/4 cups honey
1 cup unsweetened apple juice

In a bowl, sift together flour, baking soda, cinnamon, sea salt and bran. Stir in grated carrots and apples, chopped nuts and sunflower seeds. In another bowl, beat eggs, oil, honey, vanilla, apple juice, and stir into the flour mixture until the batter is just combined. Spoon batter into well greased muffin pan (or use paper cups), filling to the top and bake in preheated oven at 350 degrees for 35 to 40 minutes, or until they are well-browned on top.

✳

Nut Muffins

2 cups sifted oat flour
4 teaspoons baking powder
1/3 cup chopped nuts
1/2 teaspoon sea salt

1/4 cup rice syrup
1 egg, beaten
1/4 cup melted butter
1 cup goats milk

Sift dry ingredients together. Mix rice syrup, egg, butter and milk together thoroughly.
Combine mixtures, stirring just enough to dampen flour. Fill greased muffin pans 2/3 full.
Bake in hot oven at 400 degrees for 25 minutes.
Makes 12 to 15.

✳

Allergy-Free Muffins

1 cup rice flour	1 cup goats milk
1/2 cup oat bran	1/2 cup water
1 cut millet flour	1/2 teaspoon vanilla
1/2 teaspoon cinnamon	nut butter
1 teaspoon baking soda	fruit preserves

Preheat oven to 375 degrees. In a large bowl, mix the dry ingredients. Add the goats
milk and water, then vanilla. Mix thoroughly with spoon and pour into greased or non-
stick muffin tins. Fill cup only half full. Then add half a teaspoon or so of your favorite
fruit spread or nut butter. Fill the cups to three-fourths full. Bake for 40 minutes, or
until golden brown on top.
Makes six muffins.

✳

Corn-Rye Muffins with Cheese

1 cup rye flour	1/2 cup goats milk
1/2 cup cornmeal	1/2 cup water
2 teaspoons baking powder	1 egg
1 cup grated cheese, goats	3 tablespoons melted butter
white cheddar	

In a medium sized bowl, combine the dry ingredients well. In another bowl or a large
glass measuring cup beat together the liquid ingredients. Add the cheese to the milk
mixture and moisten thoroughly. Pour the milk-cheese mixture into the dry ingredients
and stir them quickly together. Use a minimum of strokes. Fill greased muffin pans 2/3
full. Bake at 400 degrees for 20-25 minutes, or until the crust is a beautiful golden
brown.

Blueberry Muffins

2 cups sifted oat flour
4 teaspoons baking powder
1 cup blueberries
1/2 teaspoon sea salt

1/4 cup rice syrup
1 egg, beaten
1/4 cup melted butter
1 cup goats milk

Sift dry ingredients together. Mix rice syrup, egg, butter and milk together thoroughly. Combine mixtures, stirring just enough to dampen flour. Fill greased muffin pans 2/3 full. Bake in hot oven at 400 degrees for 25 minutes.
        Makes 12 to 15.

Banana Walnut Muffins

1 1/2 cups whole-wheat
  pastry flour
2 teaspoons cinnamon
1 tablespoon baking powder
1 cup goats milk
3/4 cup chopped ripe banana

2 tablespoons honey
1 egg
2 tablespoons melted butter
1 teaspoon vanilla
1/4 cup chopped walnuts

In a medium size bowl, combine the dry ingredients and the walnuts. In another bowl, beat the liquid ingredients together with a fork. Add the banana chunks to the liquid ingredients. The banana should be chopped rather small to make sure it will be evenly distributed throughout the muffin batter. Pour the liquid ingredients and banana into the dry ingredients. Stir all together quickly with a minimum of strokes. Bake at 350 degrees for about 15-20 minutes. Center should be firm and muffins should have begun to pull away from the sides of the pan just a little.

Banana Spice Muffins
(Preheat oven to 325)

Combine: 1/2 cup goats milk
              1/2 cup rolled oats

Combine dry ingredients:

> 1 cup whole-wheat flour
> 2 1/2 teaspoons baking powder (use a no-aluminum type)
> 1/2 teaspoon baking soda
> 1/2 teaspoon sea salt
> 1/2 teaspoon cinnamon
> 1/4 teaspoon ginger
> 1/4 teaspoon nutmeg

Combine:
> 1/2 cup melted butter
> 1/4 cup honey
> 1 egg
> 1 cup bananas, mashed

With a light hand, barely combine the 3 mixtures. DO NOT BEAT. DO NOT STIR VIGOROUSLY. JUST BARELY COMBINE. A few patches of dry flour won't hurt, but over mixing will. Divide batter among 12 large, buttered muffin cups and bake 15 minutes, or until a toothpick inserted in the center of a muffin comes out clean. Remove from pan and cool 10 minutes. Serve warm.

Pineapple Bran Muffins

1 1/2 cups rice flour, sifted
3 teaspoons baking powder
1/4 cup rice syrup
1/4 cup pineapple juice
1/2 cup drained crushed pineapple
1/4 cup melted shortening

1/2 cup goats milk
1 1/2 cups bran
1 egg, beaten
1 1/4 teaspoons sea salt

Sift rice flour, baking powder and sea salt together. Add bran. Combine beaten egg, goats milk, rice syrup, pineapple juice, pineapple, crushed pineapple and shortening. Add to dry ingredients and stir just enough to dampen the rice flour. Fill greased muffin pans 2/3 full and bake in hot oven at 400 degrees for 25 minutes.

Makes 18 medium muffins.

Ginger and Pineapple Muffins

Combine:

1 cup whole-wheat pastry flour	1 tablespoon aluminum free baking powder
1/2 cup wheat germ	1/2 teaspoon sea salt
1/2 cup rolled oats	

Separately combine:

1/4 cup vegetable oil	2 eggs
1 1/2 tablespoon freshly grated ginger root	1/2 cup honey
	1 cup goats milk

Add liquid to dry ingredients stirring only to moisten. Fold in sweet pineapple, finely chopped 1/3 cup nut meats. Spoon batter into well greased muffin tin and bake 15 minutes in preheated oven. Remove muffins from tin immediately and serve warm.
    Makes 12.

Wheat-Free Poppy Fruit Muffins

Blenderize:

3 egg yolks	1/2 cup safflower oil
1 cup goats milk	1/2 cup honey

Separately Combine Dry Ingredients:

1 1/2 cups rice flour	1/2 cup oat flour
1/2 cup corn flour	1/2 teaspoon sea salt

Separate Deep Bowl:
    Beat 3 egg whites with 1 tablespoon aluminum free baking powder and set aside.

Combine blenderized and dry ingredients and mix without beating.

Fold in the egg white mixture and 1 cup finely chopped fruit in season (peaches, pears, etc.). This is a thin batter, which can be poured into the well-buttered tins. Be sure to distribute the fruits evenly throughout the muffins. Bake for 15 minutes at 375 degrees.

Makes about 16 muffins.

BREADS

Almond Bread

1 1/4 cups rice flour, sifted
1 1/2 teaspoons baking powder
1/2 cup almonds, blanched/halved
1/3 cup rice syrup

2 tablespoons lemon juice
1/8 teaspoon sea salt
4 eggs

Sift flour, baking powder and sea salt together. Beat eggs until lemon colored; add rice syrup gradually, beating constantly. Add lemon juice and shortening, continuing to beat until smooth. Add almonds and sifted dry ingredients. Pour into greased (8x8 inch) pan and bake in moderate oven at 375 degrees for 30 to 40 minutes or until well browned. Remove from pan and cut into strips or small squares.

Makes 16 (2 inch) squares.

Oatmeal-Raisin Casserole Bread

1 cup hot goats milk
1 cup oatmeal, uncooked
1 tablespoons butter
1 tablespoons virgin oil
1 teaspoon vanilla

1/4 cup maple syrup
1 cup oat flour
4 Tbs baking powder
1 tablespoon cinnamon
1/2 cup raisins

Preheat oven to 350 degrees. In a medium sized bowl, pour oatmeal and goats milk mixture into dry ingredients and mix together. Work very quickly. Mixture will foam up and you don't want to lose that rising power. Pour into a greased and oat floured 3 cup casserole dish and bake for 35 minutes, or until center tests done. Serve warm.
    Makes 6 wedges.

❈

Quick Nut Bread

1 cup chopped pecans
2 cups sifted rice flour
3 teaspoons baking powder
2 tablespoons melted shortening

1/2 cup rice syrup
1 cup goats milk
1 egg, beaten
1/2 teaspoon sea salt

Place chopped nut meats in boiling water a few minutes and drain. Sift dry ingredients together. Combine goats milk, egg, shortening and nut meats. Add to dry ingredients, mix, pour into greased loaf pan. Bake in moderate oven at 350 degrees for about 1 hour or until lightly browned.
    Makes 1 loaf.

❈

Cranberry Fruit Nut Bread

1 cup fresh or frozen
   cranberries, coarsely chopped
1/2 cup chopped nuts
1 teaspoon grated orange peel
3/4 cup orange juice
2 cups whole-wheat flour

1 cup raw sugar
1 egg, well beaten
2 tablespoons shortening
1/2 teaspoon baking soda
1 1/2 teaspoon baking
   powder

Preheat oven to 350 degrees. Generously grease lightly flour 9x3 inch loaf pan. Prepare cranberries, nuts and orange peel. Set aside. In a bowl, mix together flour, sugar, baking powder, sea salt and baking soda. Cut in shortening. Stir in orange juice, egg and orange peel, mixing just to moisten. Fold in cranberries and nuts. Spoon into prepared pan. Bake 60 minutes or until tooth pick inserted in center comes out clean. Cool on a rack 15 minutes. Remove from pan, cool completely. Wrap and store overnight.

    Makes 1 loaf.

✳

Brazil Nut-Orange Bread

3 cups sifted rice flour	1 cup sliced Brazil nuts
5 teaspoons baking powder	3/4 cup sliced orange peel
1 teaspoon sea salt	2 eggs
1 cup rice syrup	1 1/4 cups goats milk
2 tablespoons melted butter	

Quarter orange and remove peel. Scrape bitter white pulp from inside of yellow peel. Cut peel into thin slices. Cook until tender in boiling water. Drain and dry. Sift together rice flour, baking powder and sea salt. Add rice syrup, Brazil nuts and cooled orange peel. Mix well. Beat the eggs to lightness and add goats milk and melted butter. Add to dry ingredients and mix well. Put into a well-greased loaf pan and bake in a moderate oven at 350 degrees for 1 hour or until well baked.

Date Nut Bread

1 cup cut dates	1/2 teaspoon sea salt
1 cup boiling water	3/4 cup rice syrup
1 tablespoon shortening	1 egg
2 cups sifted rice flour	3 teaspoons baking powder
1 cup chopped nut meats	

Combine first 3 ingredients, cover and cool. Sift rice flour, baking powder and sea salt together. Beat rice syrup and egg together and add to dates, alternately with sifted dry ingredients. Add broken nut meats. Pour into greased loaf pan, let stand 20 minutes and

bake in slow oven at 325 degrees for 50 to 60 minutes. Turn cake on to rack to cool. The flavor of loaf improves after standing 24 hours.
 Makes 1 loaf.

✳

Nutty Banana Bread
(8 1/2" x 4 1/2" loaf)

Combine liquid ingredients:

2 ripe bananas, mashed	**1 teaspoon vanilla**
2 tablespoons cashew butter	**1 egg, beaten**
1/3 cup melted butter	**1/2 cup honey**

Combine dry ingredients:

1 1/4 cups whole-wheat (pastry flour)
1/3 cup rice flour
1/2 teaspoon sea salt
2/3 cup chopped pecans

Add dry to liquid ingredients and mix thoroughly; do not over mix. Pour the sticky mixture into a buttered and floured baking pan. Bake 60 minutes at 350 degrees. A toothpick inserted in center of bread will come out clean when bread is done. Let cool in pan 10 minutes before turning out to a wire rack. Do not slice until cool.

✳

Hominy Bread

2 cups cold cooked hominy grits	**2 eggs, separated**
1/4 teaspoon sea salt	**1 1/2 cups goats milk**
1 1/2 tablespoons melted **shortening**	

Mix hominy, sea salt and shortening. Add goats milk. Beat egg yolks thoroughly and add. Fold in egg whites beaten until stiff but not dry. Bake in greased dish in hot oven at 400 degrees for about 45 minutes.

Yellow Cornmeal Puff
(preheat oven to 350 degrees)

1 1/2 cups goats milk
3 tablespoons butter
1/2 cup yellow cornmeal
5 egg yolks
5 egg whites

1/2 teaspoon sea salt
1 cup shredded sharp,
   cheddar cheese/goats
2 tablespoons chopped
   green onion

In the top of a double boiler, cook the goats milk, butter, cornmeal and salt, stirring occasionally, until thick and steaming (about 7 minutes). Remove from heat, stir in cheese, egg yolks and green onion. Beat egg whites until stiff. Gently fold into cornmeal mixture. Turn into a well-greased 2-quart casserole. Place dish in a pan of hot water and bake in preheated oven for 35 minutes.

    Serves 6 to 8.

Cumin Corn Bread
(bean or chili dishes)

Combine:

1 cup cornmeal
1/4 cup whole-wheat flour
1/4 cup rice flour
1/4 cup wheat germ

1 teaspoon ground cumin
1 teaspoon sea salt
2 1/2 teaspoons baking
   powder

Combine in another bowl:

2 eggs, beaten
1 cup goats milk
2/3 cup cooked fresh or
   thawed frozen corn kernels

2 tablespoons honey
3 tablespoons butter,
   melted

Slowly add wet to dry ingredients until well blended. Bake in an oiled 9x9 inch baking pan for about 25 to 30 minutes at 375 degrees. Cut into squares.

Sweet Potato Puff

2 cups mashed sweet potatoes   2 tablespoons butter
sea salt/pepper to taste   1/4 cup goats milk
1 egg, separated

Combine mashed potatoes, melted butter, seasonings and goats milk. Add beaten egg yolk and beat until light and fluffy. Fold in stiffly beaten egg white. Place in buttered greased baking pan and bake at 350 degrees for 30 minutes or until puffy and browned.

*

Southern Bread

2 cups white cornmeal   3 eggs, separated
2 cups boiling water   1 1/2 cups goats milk
3 tablespoons melted shortening   1 teaspoon sea salt

Sift cornmeal 3 times and mix with boiling water, stirring until smooth and free from lumps. Add salt, shortening, goats milk and beaten egg yolks. Beat whites until stiff but not dry and fold in. Pour into greased baking dish and bake in moderate oven at 350 degrees for 45 minutes.
Serves 8.

*

Crisp Corn Bread

2 cups cornmeal   1 tablespoon butter, melted
2 cups goats milk   1 teaspoon baking powder
1 teaspoon sea salt

Mix corn meal, sea salt and baking soda together, add butter and goats milk and mix well. Pour into a depth of not over 3/4 inch in a greased shallow pan. Bake in moderate oven at 375 degrees without browning. When it begins to shrink from the sides of pan, remove from oven, brush top with melted butter and return to hot oven at 425 degrees to brown. Repeat twice in order to get brown crisp crust.
Serves 6.

Corn Bread

2 cups whole ground cornmeal	1 teaspoon baking soda
1 cup whole rice flour	2 eggs, beaten
1 teaspoon sea salt	2 cups yogurt (goats)

Rice flour combined with the cornmeal provides a natural sweetness, while the eggs and yogurt (goats) make it very moist. Combine the dry ingredients in a large bowl, then stir in the eggs and yogurt. Pour into a buttered nine-inch square pan or cast iron skillet and bake in a preheated oven at 400 degrees for 25 minutes or until golden brown.
   Serves 8.

Variations:

Add 1 cup chopped fresh pineapple or drained unsweetend, crushed pineapple.

＊

Rice and Corn bread

1 cup cornmeal (white, blue or yellow)	1 cup goats milk
2 eggs, separated	2 tablespoons olive oil
2 cups cooked brown rice	pinch sea salt
	1 cup boiling water

Put the cornmeal in a large bowl. Pour the boiling water over and let stand. Heat oven to 350 degrees. Spray a 9"x9"x2" pan with non-stick spray. Beat the egg whites until stiff, but not dry. Mix the egg yolks with the goats milk, oil and sea salt. Pour over the cornmeal and mix well. Mix the rice. Fold in the egg whites. Fold until the batter is well mixed with marble sized lumps of egg white. Pour into the prepared pan. Bake 45-50 minutes, or until the top is nicely colored and the bread has shrunk slightly away from the sides of the pan. Let cool in the pan 5 minutes before removing.
   Makes 8 2"x 4" portions.

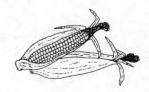

Cornmeal Batter Bread

1/2 cup cold cooked hominy	1 cup white cornmeal
1 egg, beaten	1 tablespoon butter
1 teaspoon sea salt	2 1/2 to 3 cups boiling

Mix cold hominy, egg, sea salt and cornmeal with enough boiling water to make a batter of the consistency of goats milk. Heat butter in a deep baking pan until it begins to smoke, add batter. Bake in moderate oven at 350 degrees for 40 minutes.

Makes 1 loaf.

✳

Skillet Corn Bread

4 egg yolks	1 teaspoon sea salt
4 egg whites	2 cups cornmeal
2 cups yogurt, goats	1/4 cup butter

Beat egg yolks, add yogurt, salt and cornmeal. Beat egg whites stiff and fold them into cornmeal mixture. Heat 10-inch cast-iron skilled medium hot, melt butter in it and pour in corn bread batter. Cover skilled and keep over medium hot burner for 10 minutes. Carefully loosen corn bread around the outside, cut into wedges and turn each wedge over. Cover skilled and let cook another 2 minutes or so, until top of corn bread has browned. Remove from skilled and serve hot.

Yields 8 servings.

✳

Roman Corn Bread
(preheat oven 425 degrees)

1/2 cup coarse cornmeal	1 teaspoon baking powder
1/2 cup water	3 tablespoons rice flour
1 egg	3 tablespoons melted butter

Place cornmeal in blender or food processor. Add water, egg, baking powder and rice flour, blend briefly, then add melted butter. Butter a 8x6 inch pan. Pour mixture into it and bake 10 minutes until golden. Serve at once.

Makes 15 squares.

POPOVERS, WAFERS and CRACKERS

Popovers

1 1/2 cups sifted rice flour
1/2 teaspoon sea salt

3 eggs
1 1/2 cups goats milk

Sift rice flour and sea salt. Beat eggs, add goats milk and stir gradually into rice flour to make a smooth batter. Beat thoroughly with egg beater. Fill greased custard cups or heavy metal muffin pans 2/3 full. Bake in very hot oven at 450 degrees for 15 minutes, then reduce temperature to moderate at 350 degrees and continue 20 minutes.
Makes 12 popovers.

✳

Whole-Wheat Popovers

2/3 cup sifted rice flour
1/3 cup whole-wheat flour
1 tablespoon melted shortening

2 eggs
1 cup goats milk
1/4 teaspoon sea salt

Sift rice flour and sea salt together and stir in whole-wheat flour. Combine unbeaten eggs, milk and melted shortening and add to dry ingredients. Beat well. Fill greased custard cups or heavy metal muffin pans about 1/3 full. Bake in very hot oven at 450 degrees for 25 minutes, reduce temperature to moderate at 350 degrees and bake 10 to 20 minutes longer.
Makes 8 to 10 popovers.

✳

Blender Popovers
(preheat oven 350 degrees)

Blend on high-speed 2 minutes:

1 1/2 cups goats milk
3 eggs
1/4 teaspoon sea salt
1 1/2 tablespoons melted butter

Gradually add:

1 1/2 cups whole-wheat pastry flour

Preheat oven to 450 degrees and place buttered pans in oven to preheat. Fill hot pans 2/3 full and bake 20 minutes at 450 degrees. Reduce heat to 350 degrees and bake another 15 minutes. Serve immediately or slit each popover to prevent sogginess.
Yields 12 popovers.

*

Cheese Bon-Bons

3/4 cup butter, slightly softened at room temperature
1 1/2 cup grated cheddar cheese, goats
1/4 cup grated parmesan cheese
1 1/2 cup whole-wheat pastry flour
1 tablespoon paprika
dash sea salt

In large bowl cream the butter and add the cheeses. Mix cheese and butter together thoroughly. Add the flour, salt and paprika. Mix well. Form the dough into balls about one-inch in diameter. Bake at 350 degrees for about 15 minutes.
Makes about 6 dozen.

*

Oatmeal Crackers
(preheat oven 350 degrees)

1 1/2 cup oatmeal, ground   **1/2 teaspoon sea salt**
** to a coarse flour in blender**   **5 tablespoons corn oil**
1 cup whole-wheat flour   **1 tablespoon rice syrup**

Combine dry ingredients. Combine water, oil and rice syrup (or honey). Stir dry ingredients into wet ones, to make a cohesive ball. Butter cookie sheet and pat out dough in shape of pan. Roll to thickness of 1/8 inch, using rolling pin. Score with knife in desired shapes and bake 12 minutes in preheated oven. Cool 5 minutes before removing crackers from baking sheet.
Makes 4 dozen crackers (2 inch squares).

Chive Wafers
(preheat oven 400 degrees)

1/2 cup wheat germ

1 cup whole wheat flour

1 egg

4 tablespoons chopped chives

1/4 teaspoon sea salt

1/4 cup butter

goats milk

Place wheat germ, flour and salt in a bowl. With the finger-tips or a pastry blender cut in the butter until the mixture resembles coarse oatmeal. Stir in chives, egg and enough goats milk to make a very stiff dough. Roll out the dough on a lightly floured board to 1/8 inch thickness. Cut into 1-inch rounds or fancy shapes and place on a lightly greased baking sheet. Bake in preheated oven 10 minutes or until lightly browned. Cool on a rack and store in an air-tight container.

Makes 48 wafers.

Sesame Seed Wafers
(preheat oven 400 degrees)

3 tablespoons butter, room

  temperature

1/2 cup rice flour

1/3 cup brown sugar

1/2 teaspoon vanilla

1/4 cup sesame seeds

1 egg

Place butter in a blender or food processor and combine with brown sugar. Break egg into blender or food processor, add rice flour and vanilla and blend well. Stir in sesame seeds. Drop small teaspoons of mixture onto a buttered baking sheet, leaving space for wafers to spread. Place in oven to bake for 7 minutes, until wafers spread and have lacy brown edges. They will be very thin.

Yields about 16 wafers.

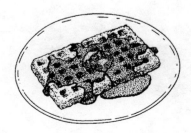

Nutty Wafers
(preheat oven 400 degrees)

1 egg
1 cup rice flour
4 tablespoons butter

1 teaspoon lemon
1/2 cup pecans, finely
2 Tbs rice syrup

Break egg into blender or food processor and blend with butter, rice syrup, rice flour and lemon juice. Stir in pecans. Place ball of dough on an ungreased baking sheet. Roll out dough to 1/8 inch thickness, and cut into 1 1/2 by 3-inch strips. Bake for 6 to 8 minutes.
     Yields 24 wafers.

※

Bran Sesame Crackers
(preheat oven to 350 degrees)

1 cup whole wheat flour
1/2 cup bran
3/4 cup oatmeal, ground to
    coarse flour in blender
1/2 teaspoon sea salt

1/2 cup water
6 tablespoons corn oil
1 tablespoon rice syrup
1/4 cup unhulled sesame seeds

Combine whole wheat, bran, oatmeal and sea salt. Combine wet ingredients and stir into dry. Grease a cookie sheet generously. Pat dough out on the cookie sheet and roll it with a rolling pin until it is as thin as possible (1/8 inch). Sprinkle sesame seeds over the surface and roll them into dough with the rolling pin. Score the dough with a knife in square or diamond shapes. Bake 10 to 12 minutes in preheated oven. Loosen crackers with a spatula as soon as they are removed from the oven. Cool and store in airtight container.
     Yields 4 dozen crackers, about 2-inch square.

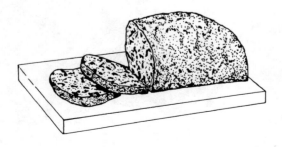

Whole Millet Cracker
(preheat oven to 350 degrees)

5 tablespoons oil
1 tablespoon honey
1/4 cup whole millet
1/2 cup millet flour

1/2 teaspoon sea salt
1/2 cup water
1 cup whole wheat flour

Combine corn oil, honey, sea salt and water. Stir in whole millet, millet flour and whole wheat flour. It may be necessary to knead dough to work in the last of the flour. Roll out dough 1/8 inch thick on buttered cookie sheet. Do not use oil as crackers may be difficult to loosen. Score crackers with a knife in square or diamond shapes, and bake in preheated oven for 20 minutes or until golden brown. Remove from cookie sheet and cool on rack.

Yields 4 dozen.

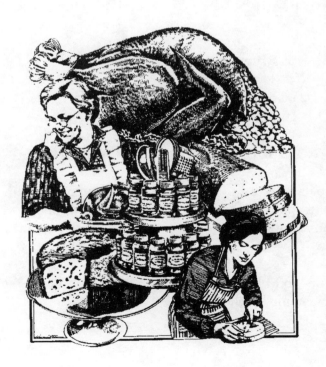

CHAPTER NINE
PARTY TIME !

Refreshments - Crepes - Desserts - Cookies
Torts - Cakes - Pies

Refreshments

Grapefruit Punch

2 lemons
3/4 cup rice syrup
2 cups water

2 1/2 cups grapefruit juice
1 1/2 cups grape juice

Slice lemons, boil with rice syrup and water 7 minutes. Cool. Add grapefruit juice and grape juice. Chill.
Makes about 1 1/2 quarts.

*

Pineapple Mint Party Punch

3 cups cold goats milk
2 cups cold pineapple juice
1 1/2 teaspoons lemon juice
3/4 cup cream

1/4 cup rice syrup
dash sea salt
12 drops peppermint
 extract

Combine all ingredients and blend until foamy. Pour into tall glasses and garnish with sprigs of mint and serve immediately.
Serves 6.

Fresh Mint Punch

12 mint sprigs, crushed
3/4 cup rice syrup
1 pint cider

3 lemons
6 oranges
3 pints ginger ale

Crush mint sprigs, squeeze the juice from the oranges and lemons over them, and add rice syrup. Stir well and then put a lump of ice in the punch bowl, pour mixture over; add cider and ginger ale.

✳

Whey Party Punch

5 cups whey
1/2 cup fresh lemon juice
2 cups fruit juice (or 2 cups
   berries)

1/4 teaspoon nutmeg
2 tablespoons fresh mint
   leaves
6 to 8 tablespoons rice
rice syrup to taste

Combine whey, lemon juice, fruit juice (or berries) in blender and process until berries are liquefied. Add nutmeg, mint and rice syrup to taste. Chill several hours before serving.
   Yields about 8 cups.

✳

Minted Strawberry/Honeydew Party Punch

16 fresh mint leaves or
 2 tablespoons dried
 peppermint tea
1 cup sliced fresh strawberries

2 tablespoons rice syrup
1 cup water
1 cup pineapple juice
1/2 honeydew, peeled and cut
   into chunks

If fresh mint leaves are not available make an infusion by pouring 1 cup boiling water over peppermint tea and allowing to steep 5 minutes. Strain and use instead of water. Combine pineapple juice, mint infusion (or water) and strawberries in blender and process until pureed. Add honeydew, rice syrup and fresh mint, if using it, and process until smooth. Chill. If you wish to serve in a punch bowl, freeze some of the punch in a small container which will fit into the punch bowl. Use this instead of ice when serving to avoid diluting punch.

Yields 4 cups.

✳

Fruit Punch

1/2 cup rice syrup	**juice 1 orange**
1 quart water	**juice 1 lemon**
1/4 teaspoon vanilla	

Cook rice syrup and water together for 10 minutes. Cool. Add fruit juices and vanilla. Makes 1 1/4 quarts. You can add leftover juices of fresh cherry, pineapple, peach or other fruits.

✳

Grapefruit Chilled

2 cups grapefruit juice	**1 1/2 cups crushed ice**
1/2 cup orange juice	**4 slices fresh lime**
dash honey, to taste	

Pour grapefruit juice, orange juice and honey into blender. Blend on high speed for about 10 seconds. Add crushed ice and blend on high for about 5 seconds. Garnish with a slice of lime.

Serves 4.

✳

Melon Milk Shake

1 medium size cantaloupe	**dash honey to taste**
1/2 cup goats milk	**1 cup vanilla ice cream**

Peel and seed cantaloupe. Cut into large chunks and place in blender. Add milk and honey and blend on high speed until melon is pureed. Add the ice cream and blend again until shake is smooth.

Serves 4.

Apricot Shake

3 tablespoons rice syrup
2 cups cold goats milk
1 cup apricot juice

1 teaspoon lemon juice
1/4 teaspoon sea salt

Dissolve rice syrup and salt in fruit juices. Chill. Before serving add to cold milk and mix well.
Serves 3.

❋

Strawberry Shake

1 egg, well beaten
1 tablespoon lemon juice

2 tablespoons rice syrup
1/2 cup crushed

Combine all ingredients and blend with chipped ice until thoroughly blended.
Serves 1.

❋

Sesame Banana Shake

2 bananas
1 tablespoon rice syrup

1 cup very cold goats milk
1 tablespoon sesame seeds

Blenderize until smooth and serve immediately.
Serves 2.

❋

Banana Milk Shake

2 fully ripe bananas

2 cups cold goats milk

Slice bananas into a bowl and beat until creamy, or press banana through coarse sieve.
Add goats milk, mix thoroughly and serve at once. Serve cold.
VARIATION:
Banana, Pineapple, Eggnog Shake
    Add 1 beaten egg and 2 tablespoons pineapple juice to above.

Frosted Apricot Milk Shake

1 cup cooked apricots and juice   3 cups goats milk
1/2 pint vanilla ice cream

Press apricots through a sieve. Mix apricot pulp and goats milk. Put ice cream in a pitcher. Pour goats milk mixture over ice cream. Stir until slightly mixed.
Serves 4 to 6.

✳

Banana Cashew Shake

1/2 cup raw cashew nuts   3 ripe bananas
1 1/2 cups water   1/8 teaspoon fresh lemon

Process cashews and water in blender. Add bananas and lemon juice and blend until bananas are liquefied. Chill and serve.
Yields 3 cups.

✳

Honey Egg Milk Shake

1 egg, well beaten   2 tablespoons honey
1 cup cold goats milk   chipped ice, optional

Combine all ingredients in a blender.
Serves 1.

✳

Eggnog

1 egg, beaten   3/4 cup goats milk
1 tablespoon rice syrup   sea salt, dash
1/4 teaspoon vanilla   nutmeg, dash

Combine egg with rice syrup and sea salt, add goats milk and vanilla. Serve cold in a tall glass and sprinkle with nutmeg.
Serve cold or hot.

VARIATION:

For a fluffy eggnog separate egg, beat white until stiff, then fold into egg yolk mixture.

✳

Nutmeg Almond Float

1/3 cup rice syrup
1/4 teaspoon nutmeg
1 teaspoon almond extract
1/2 teaspoon vanilla

1/2 teaspoon vanilla
dash sea salt
1 quart cold goats milk
1 pint vanilla ice cream

Add rice syrup, nutmeg, sea salt, almond extract, vanilla to goats milk, stir until rice syrup is dissolved. Pour into chilled glasses and top with ice cream.
Serves 6.

✳

Morning Energizer

2 cups fresh papaya juice
1 cup unsweetened pineapple juice
3 ice cubes (optional)

1 1/2 medium size bananas
 (about 1 cup)

Put all ingredients except ice cubes into blender and process until fruit is liquefied. Add ice cubes and blend a few seconds longer. Serve immediately.
Makes 4 cups.

✳

Parsley/Carrot Tonic for Two
(drink immediately after juicing)

Process through a juicer:

1 Lb carrots
2 celery stalks
6 leafy stalks parsley

Parsley/Pineapple Tonic

Liquefy thoroughly, at least one minute:

> **2 cups chilled pineapple juice, unsweetened**
> **1 cup chopped parsley**
> **5 large ice cubes**

Strain, if desired, and serve immediately with a pineapple garnish

✳

Orange Juice with Raspberries

Fill glasses with juice from chilled oranges; flat a few rasp-berries on top as a garnish.

✳

Quick Beverage

3/4 cup orange juice   **1 tablespoon rice syrup**
1 egg yolk   **1 tablespoon wheat germ**

Put all ingredients in blender and blend on high speed for about 20 seconds.
    Serves 1.

✳

Papaya Mint

1 papaya   **1/2 teaspoon fresh lemon juice**
1 1/2 cups water   **fresh mint sprigs**

Peel papaya, remove seeds and cut into pieces. Put in blender, add water and lemon juice and process until smooth. Chill and serve in parfait glasses, topped with sprig of fresh mint.
    Serves 1.

Carob Refresher
(serve hot or cold)

Carob Drink:

> **Add 2 teaspoons of *Carob Sauce to 1 cup goats milk for a carob drink.**
> *Yields 1 cup.*

*Carob Sauce:

1/3 cup honey	1 teaspoon cornstarch
1/2 cup carob	1/8 teaspoon sea salt
2/3 cup hot water	1/2 teaspoon vanilla

In a small sauce pan combine honey, carob, cornstarch, sea salt. Add water and bring to a boil, stirring constantly. Boil slowly for 5 minutes, remove from heat, cool and add vanilla. Serve hot or cold.

*

Spiced Pineapple Drink
(hot or cold)

2 cups pineapple juice	**1 stick cinnamon**
6 to 8 cloves	

Combine ingredients, heat slowly to boiling, strain and serve hot or cold.
Serves 1.

*

Oranges and Strawberries with Honey

1 medium orange	**1 tablespoon alfalfa honey**
1/2 cup strawberries, fresh or frozen without sugar	

Peel and slice orange, top with strawberries and drizzle with honey.
Serves 1.

Orange/Grape Juice Fluff

3 tablespoons orange juice
1/2 cup grape juice
1 egg white, stiffly beaten

2 teaspoons rice syrup
dash sea salt

Combine fruit juices. Beat egg white until frothy, add rice syrup and sea salt and beat until stiff. Stir egg white carefully into fruit juices.
Serves 1.

✳

Orange Slushy

1 large can frozen orange juice concentrate
1 tray ice cubes, crushed
orange peel and mint sprigs (optional)

Mix concentrate and crushed ice in blender. Blend on high until thoroughly mixed. Garnish with a twist of orange peel and a sprig of mint.
Serves 4.

✳

Pineapple-Carrot Beverage

1 3/4 cups unsweetened
  pineapple with juice
2 large carrots, washed,
  scraped and cut into
  1-inch pieces

1/4 inch slice of lemon
  juice
1 cup water

Combine all ingredients in blender and process to a thick, shrub consistency.
Makes 4 cups.

✳

Orange Nog

2 cups goats milk
1 tablespoon rice syrup
honey egg milk shake

1 cup orange juice
2 teaspoons grated orange
  rind

Place goats milk and rice syrup in blender. Add orange juice and rind and blend. If orange juice is very tart add more rice syrup.

Serves 2.

✳

Creamy Nog

3 oranges	1 egg
1 small banana	4 ice cubes
1/2 cup vanilla yogurt, goats	orange slices for garnish

Cut oranges into halves and extract juice; measure one cup juice. Place orange juice, banana, yogurt, egg and ice cubes in a blender or food processor. Cover, process until smooth. Pour into serving glasses and garnish with orange slices.

Serves 2.

✳

Yogurt Smoothies

2 cups plain yogurt, goats	1/2 cup pineapple juice
2 ripe bananas	6 ice cubes, crushed

Place all ingredients in blender and whirl until smooth. Serve in champagne glasses, topped with a dusting of nutmeg, if desired.

✳

Tomato Beverage

4 cups cooked tomatoes	3 tablespoons lemon juice
1 teaspoon grated lemon rind	1/2 teaspoon sea salt
few drops Worcestershire sauce	

Press tomatoes through sieve, add remaining ingredients and chill. Shake or stir well before serving.

Serves 4 to 6.

Tomato Smoothie

1 1/2 cup tomato juice
1/2 cup yogurt, goats
1 teaspoon Spike
6 to 10 drops hot sauce

Put all ingredients, except parsley, into blender in the order listed. Blend until smooth. Tomato juice may be chilled first, if desired.
Serves 2.

✳

Tomato Flip

4 cups tomato juice	1/4 cup chopped parsley
1/4 onion, chunked	4 thin celery sticks
1/2 cup green pepper, chunked	4 lemon slices
dash Worcestershire sauce	juice from 1 lemon

Put in blender tomato juice, chunks of onion and green pepper, lemon juice, parsley and Worcestershire sauce. Blend on high-speed until smooth. Chill. Stir before serving. Pour into 4 tall glasses. Add a celery "swizzle stick" to each glass. Float a slice of lemon on top and serve.
Serves 4.

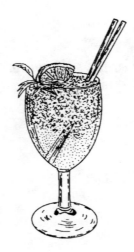

CREPES
(Fillings/Sauces)

Standard Method for Cooking Crepes

Heat heavy skillet or crepe pan to medium-high heat. Pan is ready when a drop of water "dances" on it. Oil pan well, stir batter, then our it into pan. 1/4 cup batter will make about the right size crepe. Add more goats milk, if necessary, to make a thin crepe. Let crepe cook approx. 2 minutes. It should be golden brown underneath and dry on top. Flip crepe over and let second side brown for approx. 1 minute. Slide crepe onto heat proof plate and keep warm in low oven until ready to fill and serve. Crepes may be stacked on top of each other.

Oatmeal Crepes

4 eggs	1 tablespoon rice syrup
2 cups goats milk	2 tablespoons butter
1 1/2 cups oat flour	1/2 teaspoon sea salt

Combine all ingredients in blender and process until batter is smooth. Let rest for 2 hours to allow particles of flour to expand in liquid, resulting in a tender crepe. Just before baking crepes, process again briefly to blend ingredients.

Crepes Suzette (Second phase)

4 eggs	1 cup goats milk
1 tablespoon rice syrup	1 3/4 cups whole-wheat
2 tablespoons melted butter	pastry flour
1/2 teaspoon sea salt	1 cup water

Combine first seven ingredients in blender and process until batter is smooth. Let stand for 2 hours to allow particles of flour to expand in liquid, resulting in a tender crepe. Just before baking crepes, process batter again briefly to blend ingredients.

Apricot Crepe Sauce (Second phase)

1/2 cup dried apricots
1/4 cup rice syrup

2 slices lemon, including
1 cup rind

Combine all ingredients in a small saucepan and cook slowly for about 20 minutes. Cool, then puree in blender. Serve hot or cold.

Yields approx. 1 cup.

Quick Crepes

1/2 cup rice flour, scant
2 tablespoons unsalted butter,
  melted

1/2 cup water plus
2 tablespoons water
1 egg

Combine the above ingredients in blender or food processor. Use a 7-inch diameter crepe pan. Place over medium-high heat. Rub a drop of butter on bottom of pan with a paper towel, but do not butter pan heavily as butter will burn. When pan is hot, a drop of water will dance. Pour 2 tablespoons batter into hot pan, tilting pan so that it spreads evenly into a thin pancake. Lower heat to medium. Cook until bubbles form and crepe is lightly browned, about 1 or 2 minutes; turn and cook about 1 minute. Make crepes as needed as batter keeps well if refrigerated.

Makes 10 crepes.

Zucchini Puree for Quick Crepes

4 small zucchini
1/4 cup yogurt, goats

paprika
cayenne pepper

Place zucchini in blender or food processor and puree. Place puree in a bowl and stir in goat yogurt and season to taste with paprika and cayenne pepper.

Yields about 1 cup.

Cranberry Crepe Yogurt Sauce

1/4 cup cranberry puree	1/2 cup yogurt, goats
1/4 cup honey	1/4 cup softened butter

Combine all ingredients. Using blender make a puree. Serve with crepes or pancakes.
Yields 1 1/4 cups.

✳

Party Pancakes
(brunch or luncheon)

1 cup minced cooked chicken or turkey	1/2 teaspoon sea salt
1 tablespoons butter	dash pepper
1 tablespoon rice flour	1/2 teaspoon tarragon
1 cup yogurt, goats	2 tablespoons melted butter
1 small white onion, minced	parmesan cheese

Cook the onion in 1 tablespoon butter. Add second tablespoon butter and sprinkle with the rice flour, stir well. Add the chicken and the yogurt; cover and simmer gently until needed, stirring occasionally. Add tarragon and spread this mixture on the pancakes; roll them up and place in a buttered casserole or shallow Pyrex dish. Pour over them a little melted butter, sprinkle with Parmesan cheese, and put under broiler 2 or 3 minutes to brown. The pancakes may also be arranged on a layer of spinach puree or topped with a cranberry sauce.

✳

Spinach Puree for Party Pancakes

3 Lbs fresh spinach	dash sea salt
1 tablespoon rice flour	dash pepper
1/2 teaspoon minced onion	dash nutmeg
little yogurt, goats	

Pick over spinach (about 3 Lbs) and remove coarse stems and roots. Wash thoroughly in several waters and cook covered, in own juice, no longer than 10 minutes (or less if spinach is very young or fresh). Add sea salt at the last. Drain and chop fine and press out the water, which should be kept for soup. Cook in a saucepan butter, rice flour and minced onion. Add the chopped spinach, stir well and add dash of nutmeg, pepper and a little yogurt and reheat.

✳

Rice and Soy Crepes
(with Sprouts/avocado Crepe filling)

4 eggs
2 tablespoons sesame oil
2 cups water

1 cup brown rice flour
1/2 cup soy flour
1/2 teaspoon sea salt

Combine all ingredients in blender and process until batter is smooth. Let rest for 2 hours to allow particles of flour to expand in liquid, resulting in a tender crepe. Just before baking crepes, process again briefly to blend ingredients. Follow standard method for cooking crepes and serve with Sprouts/Avocado Crepe Filling (see below).
Yields 12 8-inch crepes.

✳

Sprouts/Avocado Crepe Filling

2 ripe medium-size avocados,
  peeled and pitted
1 cup mung bean sprouts
3 tablespoons lemon juice

1 clove garlic, minced
pepper
sea salt
1/4 cup sesame seed butter

Mash avocados and combine with all ingredients, except sprouts, to make filling. Put 2 tablespoons filling and 1 tablespoon sprouts on each crepe. Roll or fold crepe and serve.
Fills approximately 16 8-inch crepes.

✳

Crepe Filling Sauce

2 tablespoons butter
3/4 chopped green pepper
1/2 cup chopped onion
2 medium ripe tomatoes, peeled
  and chopped

1/4 teaspoon oregano
1/4 teaspoon freshly ground
pepper

Melt butter in skillet. Cook and stir green pepper and onion until in butter until onion is tender. Stir in remaining ingredients. Cover and simmer 5 minutes.

Serves 4.

✳

Tiny Cream Puffs
(preheat oven to 400 degrees)

1 cup water	1/4 teaspoon sea salt
1/2 cup butter	1 cup whole-wheat flour
4 eggs	

Bring water, butter and sea salt to a boil in a medium-size saucepan. Remove pan from heat. Add whole-wheat flour all at once, stirring hard with a wooden spoon. Lower heat and continue to cook dough, stirring constantly, for a minute or two to make sure flour is cooked. Transfer dough to bowl of electric mixer. Add eggs, one at a time, beating well after each addition. Drop dough by teaspoon onto a lightly buttered cookie sheet, leaving 1 inch between each puff. Bake in preheated oven for 25 to 30 minutes or until they are quite firm. Loosen carefully with spatula and cool on wire rack. Store in a cool dry place until time to split and fill them. Filling should be done just before serving to prevent them from getting soggy.

Makes approximately 6 dozen 1 1/2-inch puffs.

✳

Boiled Custard Sauce

2 eggs, slightly beaten	1/2 teaspoon sea salt
1/4 cup rice syrup	1/2 teaspoon vanilla
2 cups goats milk, scaled	

Combine eggs, sea salt and sugar; add goats milk slowly and cook in top of double boiler until mixture coats a spoon. Add vanilla and turn into individual serving dishes and chill.

Serves 4.

Baked Orange Custard

4 eggs, separated   1 cup rice syrup
1/2 cup orange juice   1 tablespoon grated orange

Beat egg yolks until light; add rice syrup slowly, beating constantly. Add orange juice and rind., When well mixed fold in stiffly beaten egg whites. Pour into greased baking dish, place in pan of hot water and bake at 350 degrees about 35 minutes or until firm. Serve immediately with fresh fruit or dessert sauce.
    Serves 6.
VARIATION:
        Lemon: Use 3 tablespoons lemon juice
                      and 1 teaspoon grated lemon
                      rind instead of orange.

✳

Thick Custard

2 1/2 tablespoons cornstarch   1 cup goats milk
1/2 teaspoon vanilla extract   2 tablespoons rice syrup
2 egg yolks

Dissolve cornstarch in a little of the cold milk. Heat remaining milk in top of double boiler. Stir dissolved cornstarch into hot milk and cook until thickened, stirring constantly. Beat egg yolks with rice syrup. Stir a little of the hot milk into the egg mixture and stir this into the remaining hot milk. Cook for approximately 1 minute, stirring constantly. Add vanilla extract. Pour into container and chill.
    Yields 1 1/4 cups.

✳

Banana Tapioca Cream Dessert

2 tablespoons quick-cooking   1/4 teaspoon sea salt
1/3 cup rice syrup   2 cups scaled goats milk
1 egg, separated   1 teaspoon grated orange
1 cup diced ripe bananas

Mix tapioca, sea salt and half the rice syrup together. Add goats milk and cook over boiling water about 5 minutes, or until tapioca is clear, stirring frequently. Combine egg yolk and remaining rice syrup. Add a small amount of the tapioca mixture, stirring constantly. Then pour back into remaining hot mixture beating vigorously. Continue cooking about 5 minutes, stirring constantly. Fold in beaten egg white. Cool. Add orange rind and bananas. Chill. Garnish with sliced ripe bananas.

Serves 6.

✳

Lemon Tapioca Fluff

2 tablespoons quick-cooking tapioca	1 egg yolk
2 tablespoons rice syrup	1 egg white
2 tablespoons honey	1 cup fresh lemon juice
	1 teaspoon grated lemon peel

Mix tapioca, 2 tablespoons rice syrup and the lemon peel in saucepan. Blend in egg yolk and lemon juice; let stand 5 minutes. Cook over medium heat, stirring constantly, just until mixture boils. Remove from heat. Beat egg whites, until foamy. Beat in 2 tablespoons honey, 1 tablespoon at a time; beat until stiff and glossy. Do not underbeat. Fold in tapioca mixture and cool. Divide among 3 dessert dishes and refrigerate.

Serves 3.

✳

New Mexican Pudding
(preheat oven 300 degrees)

3 cups goats milk	3 tablespoons honey
1/4 cup butter	2/3 cup rice syrup
2/3 cup cornmeal	1 teaspoon sea salt
3/4 teaspoon cinnamon	3/4 teaspoon nutmeg
1 cup goats milk	

Heat 3 cups goats milk. Stir in butter, rice syrup and honey. Combine cornmeal, sea salt cinnamon and nutmeg and stir gradually into warm milk mixture, using a wire whisk to avoid lumps. Cook over low heat, stirring constantly, approx. 10 minutes or until thick.

Turn into oiled casserole, pour 1 cup goats milk over pudding (do not stir), and bake in preheated oven for 3 hours.

✳

Blueberry Pudding (Full of Life phase)
(preheat oven 325 degrees)

2 egg yolks
1/4 cup rice syrup
2 tablespoons soft butter
1 cup of papaya juice
1 cup fresh blueberries
  (or raspberries)

1/4 teaspoon cinnamon
2 egg whites, stiffly
  beaten
1 1/2 cups soft rye bread
  crumbs

Beat egg yolks and rice syrup together. Add soft butter and beat in to blend. Add papaya juice, bread crumbs, cinnamon and blueberries. Carefully fold in stiffly beaten egg whites. Pour into ungreased casserole dish and bake in preheated oven for 45 minutes or until set. Cool slightly and serve pudding warm with yogurt (goats).
  Serves 4.

✳

Potato Pudding
(preheat oven 350 degrees)

1 medium potato, pared
1/4 teaspoon grated lemon peel
1 egg white

2 tablespoons butter
1 tablespoon rice syrup

Cut potato into quarters. Heat 1 inch water (do not add salt) to boiling. Add potatoes; cover and heat to boiling. Cook until tender, 20 to 25 minutes. Drain. Heat oven to 350 degrees. Grease 2 1/2 cup casserole with butter. Mash potatoes until no lumps remain. Beat in lemon peel, butter and rice syrup. Beat egg white until stiff. Fold potato mixture into egg white. Turn into casserole. Bake uncovered until golden brown, approx. 25 minutes.
  Serves 2.

Blueberry Yogurt Dessert (Full of Life phase)

1 cup fresh or frozen blueberries, thawed/drained
3 small oranges (approx. 1 Lb
  peeled, seeded and cut into
  chunks)

1 tablespoon honey
10 tablespoons yogurt,
  goats

Put oranges in blender and process to a liquid. Then add blueberries and blend to a liquid. Add honey and yogurt and process to combine. Pour into serving dishes and chill.

  Yields approx. 3 cups.

Almond Cream Dessert

5 egg whites
3/4 cup rice syrup

1 teaspoon vanilla
3/4 cup grated almonds

Beat the egg whites until stiff, add 1/2 cup rice syrup, and then gently fold in the remaining cup. Add the vanilla and gently fold in the almonds (grate in blender). This should be cold, but since it must be done at the last minute, keep ingredients in refrigerator until you are ready to make it. Serve in sherbet glasses.

Baked Hawaiian Peach Dessert (Full of Life phase)

8 firm medium peaches
1/2 cup canned unsweetened pineapple juice

1/2 cup rice syrup

Pour boiling water over peaches. Rub off skins and place peaches close together in baking dish. Pour rice syrup over peaches, add pineapple juice, cover and bake at 350 degrees for about 20 minutes. Remove cover and brown fruit slightly. Serve hot or cold.

  Serves 8.

Banana Dessert

6 firm bananas   3/4 cup maple syrup
2 tablespoons lemon juice   1/4 cup chopped pecans

Peel bananas, brush with lemon juice and place in greased baking dish. Pour maple syrup over bananas. Bake at 375 degrees for 15 to 18 minutes. Sprinkle with nuts.
Serves 6.

Creamy Rice Dessert

1/2 cup rice   1 tablespoon rice syrup
2 or 3 cups goats milk   nutmeg or cinnamon
dash sea salt

Wash rice well and cook in double boiler until soft or about 1 1/2 hours, stirring occasionally. Add a little more milk if necessary, as it should be creamy and not stiff when cold. Pour into a bowl or shallow dish and sprinkle with a little nutmeg or cinnamon.

✳

Crushed Fruit Tapioca

1/2 cup Minute tapioca   1 tablespoon lemon
1/4 cup water   3 1/2 cups crushed fruit
1 teaspoon butter   strawberries, raspberries, etc.)
3/4 cup rice syrup   dash sea salt

Crush the fruit and let stand with the rice syrup long enough to draw the juice. Put the tapioca, water, sea salt, butter, and juice drained from the fruit into a double boiler, stir well, and cook until clear. Add fruit, pour into a glass serving dish and chill.

Vanilla Dessert Sauce

1/2 cup rice syrup
1 tablespoon cornstarch
1 cup boiling water

2 tablespoons butter
1 teaspoon vanilla
few grains sea salt

Mix rice syrup and cornstarch; add water gradually, stirring constantly. Boil for 5 minutes, remove from heat, add butter, vanilla and sea salt. Stir until butter is melted and serve hot.

Makes approx. 1 cup sauce.

✳

Butterscotch Dessert Sauce

1/4 cup butter
1/2 cup yogurt, goats
dash sea salt

1 cup brown sugar
   (Sucanat)
2 eggs separated

Cream butter and sugar. Beat yolks until thick, add yogurt; beat into butter and sugar mixture. Cook in top of double boiler until thickened. Pour slowly over salted egg whites, beaten until stiff but not dry. Serve hot.

Makes 2 1/2 cups sauce.

✳

Caramel Dessert Sauce

1 cup Sucanat
1/2 cup boiling water

2 tablespoons yogurt, goats

Place rice syrup in heavy pan and heat slowly until melted and browned, stirring constantly. Add boiling water slowly, stirring vigorously. Cook until syrup and all of Sucanat has melted. Remove from heart and add cream. Serve hot or cold. If too thick when cold, add a little more yogurt.

Makes about 1 cup.

Raspberry Sauce Melba
(ice cream, sherbet or fruits)

1 package (10 ounce) frozen
   raspberries thawed

1/4 cup rice syrup
1/2 teaspoon vanilla

Place all ingredients in blender and blend on high speed about 30 seconds. If desired, pour sauce into refrigerator tray and freeze until firm.
> *Yields about 1 1/3 cups.*

✳

Fruit Dessert Sauce

2 tablespoons cornstarch
2 tablespoons water
1/2 teaspoon lemon juice

1 cup crushed pineapple
2 tablespoons rice syrup

Mix cornstarch and water in small saucepan. Stir in pineapple. Cook, stirring constantly, until mixture thickens and boils, Remove from heat, stir in rice syrup and lemon juice. Cover and refrigerate at least 1 hour.
> *Yields 1 cup.*

✳

Cherry Dessert Sauce

1/4 cup rice syrup
2 tablespoons rice flour
1 cup hot red cherry juice

1/4 cup butter
2 tablespoons lemon juice
2 drops almond extract

Combine rice syrup and rice flour, stir in cherry juice gradually, heat to boiling and cook until thickened, stirring constantly. Add butter, lemon juice and almond extract. Serve hot or cold.
> *Makes 1 1/4 cups.*

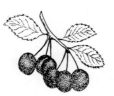

Cranberry Sauce

1 1/2 cups rice syrup   1 Lb (4 cups) cranberries
2 cups water

Boil rice syrup and water together 5 minutes. Add cranberries and boil without stirring until all skins pop open; about 5 minutes. Remove from heat and cool.
Makes 4 cups sauce.

✳

Sunflower Seed Cookies
(preheat oven to 275 degrees)

2 egg whites   1/4 cup honey
1 cup sunflower seeds   1 teaspoon vanilla
   (ground to a meal in blender)

Beat egg whites until stiff, then gradually beat in honey and vanilla. Carefully fold in sunflower seed meal. Drop batter by teaspoon onto a well-buttered cookie sheet and bake in preheated oven for 30 minutes. Loosen cookies from baking sheet as soon as possible after removing them from oven. They will be a bit soft to the touch but will harden as they cool. Store in air-tight container.
Makes 2 dozen cookies.

✳

Quick Almond Oatmeal Cookies

1 1/2 sticks butter   1/2 teaspoon baking soda
1 cup rice syrup   1 teaspoon sea salt
1/4 cup water   1 teaspoon almond extract
2 cups Quick Quaker Oats   1/2 cup finely chopped
1 cup rice flour   blanched almonds

Mix the butter, rice syrup, water and almond extract and beat until smooth. Sift the dry ingredients together and add to the creamy mixture. Add the Quick Quaker Oats and the almonds. Drop by the teaspoon onto greased cookie sheets and slightly press down. Bake 14 minutes at 350 degrees

Almond Cookies
(preheat oven 375 degrees)

1/2 cup almonds
2 tablespoons butter
1 teaspoon almond or
   vanilla extract

1 tablespoon rice flour
2 tablespoons goats milk
1/4 cup rice syrup

Place almonds in food processor or blender and grind fine. Add butter, rice syrup and blend with almonds. Add rice flour, goats milk and almond (or vanilla) extract and mix well. Drop batter by teaspoons in small rounds onto a buttered baking sheet. Bake for 4 to 5 minutes.
   Yields 12 small cookies.

✳

Banana Pecan Cookies (Full of Life phase)

2 1/4 cups rice flour
2 teaspoons baking powder
1/4 teaspoon baking soda
2 eggs, beaten
1/2 teaspoon vanilla

1 cup rice syrup
1/2 teaspoon sea salt
1/3 cup shortening
1 cup mashed bananas
1/2 cup chopped pecans

Sift together dry ingredients. Cream shortening and rice syrup thoroughly, add eggs, vanilla and beat well. Add banana alternately with dry ingredients. Stir in chopped pecans. Drop by teaspoons onto greased cookie sheet and bake at 350 degrees 15 minutes.
   Makes about 60 cookies.

✳

Orange Cookies
(preheat oven to 400 degrees)

3 tablespoons butter
1/2 cup rice flour
1 teaspoon baking powder

2 tablespoons fresh orange
   juice
2 tablespoons rice syrup

Place butter, rice flour and baking powder in blender or food processor and blend. Add fresh orange juice and rice syrup and mix to combine. Place teaspoonfuls of batter on a buttered baking sheet. Bake for 6 to 7 minutes.

Yields 8 cookies.

*

Almond and Tahini Cookies

2 eggs
1/2 cup tahini
1 1/2 teaspoons baking powder
4 tablespoons butter

1 cup rice syrup
1 teaspoon vanilla
2 cups rice flour
1/2 cup blanched almonds, pulverized

Place all the ingredients except the rice flour in a food processor and process for a few moments, then transfer to a mixing bowl. Add the flour and knead into a dough, then form into balls about 1" in diameter. Flatten to about 1/4" thickness on well greased cookie sheets and bake in a preheated 350 degree oven for 15 minutes. Cool before serving or storing.

Makes about 3 1/2 dozen cookies.

*

Sesame Cookies
(preheat oven to 350 degrees)

1 cup sesame seeds
3/4 cup corn oil
1 cup rice syrup
1/2 teaspoon vanilla or
  almond extract

1/2 teaspoon baking soda
1 teaspoon baking powder
2 cups rice flour

Spread sesame seeds on a baking sheet and toast them lightly. Cream the oil and rice syrup and gradually sift in the dry ingredients. Add the vanilla (or almond extract) and mix in the sesame seeds. Bake on an oiled cookie sheet about 12 minutes at 350 degrees.

Carob Nut Brownies
(preheat oven to 350 degrees)

2 eggs, beaten

1/2 cup honey

1/4 teaspoon almond extract

1 cup whole wheat pastry flour

2/3 cup chopped walnuts

1 tablespoon rice syrup

1/4 melted butter

1 cup carob, sifted

1/2 teaspoon sea salt

Combine eggs, honey, rice syrup, butter and almond extract. Mix rice flour, carob and sea salt, then combine the wet and dry mixtures. Mix thoroughly, add walnuts and turn into an oiled 8x8 inch baking pan. Bake in preheated oven for 25 minutes. Remove from oven and cut while warm. Cool on rack.

Yield 16 brownies.

Carob Walnut Brownies
(Preheat oven to 350 degrees)

2 eggs, beaten

1/2 cup honey

1 tablespoon rice syrup

1/4 cup melted butter

1/4 teaspoon almond extract

1 cup whole wheat pastry
  flour

1 cup carob, sifted

1/2 teaspoon sea salt

2/3 cup chopped walnuts

Combine eggs, honey, butter and almond extract. Mix four, carob and sea salt, then combine the wet dry mixtures. Mix thoroughly, add nuts and turn into an oiled 8x8 inch baking pan. Bake in preheated oven for about 25 minutes. Remove from oven and cut while warm. Cool on rack.

Yields 16 brownies.

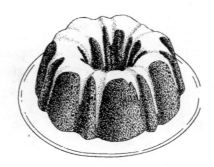

Carob Honey Cake
(preheat oven to 350 degrees)

1 cup whole wheat pastry flour
1/2 cup carob, sifted
2 teaspoons cinnamon
6 egg yolks
6 egg whites, stiffly beaten

1/3 cup softened butter
1/2 cup honey
1/3 cup water
2 teaspoons vanilla

Combine flour, carob and cinnamon. Mix well. Beat egg yolks with butter and honey. Add water and vanilla. Combine dry and wet mixtures and mix thoroughly, then fold in beaten egg whites. Turn into a buttered 9 inch spring-form pan and bake for approx. 40 minutes in preheated oven. Frost with Carob Nut Frosting (see below), if desired.

✳

Carob Nut Frosting

3 tablespoons honey
3 tablespoons softened butter
4 tablespoons cottage cheese
    (pureed in blender until smooth)

1/3 cup carob, sifted
1/2 cup chopped nuts
2/3 cup goats dry milk

In electric mixer, beat honey and butter together, then stir in goats dry milk and carob. Add pureed cottage cheese, mixing until smooth. Spread over cake and top with chopped nuts.
Yield: frosting to cover 1 9-inch loaf cake or 2 8-inch layers.

✳

Party Walnut Torte
(preheat oven to 350 degrees)

2 cups walnuts
4 egg whites
4 egg yolks

6 tablespoons honey
1 teaspoon vanilla

Grind walnuts, 1/2 cut at a time in blender. Beat egg whites until stiff, then set aside. Beat egg yolks, then beat in honey and vanilla, and finally, mix in ground nuts. Fold in beaten egg whites carefully, then turn batter into greased 9x9 inch pan or a 9-inch layer cake pan. Bake for 10 minutes in preheated oven. Then turn oven down to 325 degrees and continue to bake for approximately 25 minutes longer or until cake tests done when an inserted toothpick comes out clean. Cool for 10 minutes then remove from pan if desired. Serve warm or cold with a fruit sauce.

✳

Carrot Torte

8 eggs, separated	grated rind 1 orange
2 cups rice syrup	1 Lb carrots, cooked and grated
1 Lb almonds, blanched and chopped fine	

Beat egg yolks until thick, beat in rice syrup gradually, then add juice and rind of orange. Add carrots and nuts. Fold in stiffly beaten egg whites. Bake in greased torte pan at 350 degrees for 50 minutes.

✳

Sunshine Cake

2 cups sifted rice flour	1 cup cornmeal
4 1/2 teaspoons baking powder	3 eggs, beaten
1 cup goats milk	1/2 cup maple syrup
3/4 cup melted shortening	3/4 teaspoon sea salt

Sift rice flour, baking powder and sea salt together, add cornmeal and mix thoroughly. Combine remaining ingredients and add to dry ingredients, stirring only enough to dampen all the flour. Pour into greased pan and bake in hot oven (400 degrees) 30 minutes.

Serves 8.

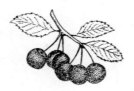

Spice Cake
(with Quick Caramel Frosting)

1 cup rice syrup
1 cup water
1/3 cup butter
2 cups cake rice flour
1 teaspoon double-acting baking powder

good pinch nutmeg
1/2 teaspoon cinnamon
1/2 teaspoon allspice
1/2 cup chopped almonds

Boil the water, margarine, rice syrup, and spices 3 minutes. Allow to cool. Sift the flour and baking powder twice and remeasure. Stir gradually into the boiled mixture, and when smooth add the chopped nuts. Bake in a greased tub pan 1 hour in a pre-heated 325 degree oven.

✳

Quick Caramel Frosting

2 cups rice syrup
1 teaspoon vanilla

1/3 cup water
3 tablespoons butter

Stir until dissolved, cover and cook 3 minutes, uncover and cook without stirring until it forms a ball in cold water. Add the butter and let cool slightly Add the vanilla and beat until thick and creamy.

✳

Oat Flour Pie Crust

Oat flour makes a light, crisp pie crust and the dough is very easy to handle. Amount of water is variable here, add enough to make a smooth, workable dough. No need to chill it.

4 tablespoons butter, cold
1 cup oat flour

1/2 cup ice water

Chop butter into pieces and pour flour over. Rub with your fingers until the butter and flour resemble coarse meal, just like regular pie crust. Begin adding ice water, a little at a time, until a smooth pliable dough is formed. Roll out using more oat flour and proceed as for regular pie crust. Bake at 325 degrees for about 20 minutes and then fill it with a prepared filling to prevent sogginess of the bottom of the crust.

✳

Plain Pastry
(preheat oven 400 degrees)

2 cups rice flour, sifted   **2/3 cup corn oil**
3/4 teaspoon sea salt   **4 to 6 tablespoons cold water**

Sift rice flour and sea salt and corn oil. Add water, using only a small portion at a time until mixture will hold together. Divide dough into 2 parts. Roll out on floured board to desired size. Line the pie pan with one piece of dough, being careful not to stretch dough. After filling is placed in pastry, dampen edges of lower crust with cold water and cover with remaining dough which has been rolled out and slashed several places to allow steam to escape while baking. Press edges together with prongs of fork and bake according to recipe for filling selected.

Makes 2 (9-inch) pie shells or one 2-crust (9-inch) pie.

✳

Basic Pie Crust
(preheat oven 400 degrees)

1 cup blue corn pastry flour   **3 to 4 teaspoons ice water**
1/4 cup softened butter   **1/4 teaspoon sea salt**

Mix sea salt and flour together, then cut butter in with a fork and knife or pastry cutter. Add the water slowly until dough forms a ball. Do not overwork. Roll out on a lightly floured surface to about 12 inches in diameter. Carefully lift one side, fold it in half, and lift into the pie plate, centering the fold in the middle of the pan. Unfold and trim away the excess or flute the edges. If you need to bake the crust before filling, bake at 400 degrees for 10 to 15 minutes. Prick the bottom with a fork before baking to prevent air bubbles.

Makes one pie crust.

Whole Wheat & Walnut Pastry Pie Shell (second phase)
(preheat oven to 375 degrees)

1/4 cup ground walnuts	1/4 teaspoon sea salt
1 cup whole wheat pastry flour	1/4 cup corn oil
1/4 cup wheat germ	2 tablespoons cold water

Combine nuts, flour, wheat germ, sea salt and corn oil. Add cold water gradually, tossing mixture gently to distribute evenly. Press into a 9-inch pie pan. Bake in preheated oven for approximately 15 minutes or until nicely brown.

Oat and Rice Flaky Pastry (second phase)
(preheat oven to 400 degrees)

3/4 cup oat flour	1/2 teaspoon sea salt
3/4 cup brown rice flour	1 tablespoon corn oil
6 tablespoons butter	2 tablespoons ice water

Sprinkle a 9-inch pie pan lightly with flour. Combine flours and sea salt in a bowl. Cut butter in with knives or a grater. Add corn oil gradually, working it in with fingers, then the ice water. Knead dough briefly until water is distributed evenly. Press into prepared pie pan or roll out between well-floured sheets of was paper and place in pie pan, make a high fluted edge around the outside. If baking shell without filling, prick it well with a fork. Bake in preheated oven for 10 to 12 minutes.

Makes 1 9-inch pie shell.

Walnut Pie (second phase)

For filling combine:

3 eggs, beaten	1 1/2 cups rice syrup
2/3 teaspoon sea salt	1 1/2 tablespoon whole-
3/4 cup honey	wheat pastry flour
1/2 cup butter, melted	

Mix well, then add:

1 1/2 cups chopped walnuts   1 1/2 teaspoon lime juice
3/4 teaspoon vanilla extract

Pour filling into unbaked crust and bake in preheated 350 degrees oven for 30 minutes on low oven rack. Reduce heat to 300 degrees and bake 15 minutes longer, checking carefully to prevent burning. Cool pie thoroughly on a rack and chill before serving.
    Makes one 9 1/2"-10" pie.

✳

Cranberry Pie
(preheat oven 450 degrees)

4 cups cranberries   1 1/2 cups rice syrup
2 tablespoons rice flour   1/4 teaspoon sea salt
3 tablespoons water   1 tablespoon melted butter
1 recipe plain pastry

Wash cranberries, chop and mix with rice syrup, rice flour, sea salt and water. Line pie pan with pastry, pour filling. Bake in very hot oven (450 degrees) for 15 minutes and reduce to moderate, 350 degrees and bake about 30 minutes longer.
    Makes 1 9-inch pie.

✳

Pumpkin Pie
(Basic Pie Crust)

1 unbaked basic pie crust   1 cup dry goats milk powder
1/2 teaspoon cinnamon   1/8 teaspoon allspice
1 1/2 cup cooked pumpkin, pureed   1 tablespoon rice syrup
3 eggs beaten   1/4 teaspoon sea salt
1 cup water   1/2 teaspoon ground ginger
1/3 cup honey   1 teaspoon cinnamon
1/4 teaspoon nutmeg

Prepare Basic Pie Crust according to directions (see below), adding 1/2 teaspoon cinnamon to the flour mixture BEFORE the ice water is added. Combine the pumpkin, honey, rice syrup, and eggs and mix until smooth. Stir in the spices, water and dry goats milk powder until well-blended. Pour the pumpkin mixture into the prepared, unbaked pie crust and bake in a preheated oven at 425 degrees for 15 minutes. Then turn the heat down to 350 degrees and continue to bake for 1 hour, or until a knife inserted in the center comes out clean. Allow to cool completely, then cover and refrigerate.

✳

Blackberry Pie
(preheat 450 degrees)

3 cups fresh blackberries	2 tablespoons lemon juice
1 cup rice syrup	1/8 teaspoon sea salt
2 tablespoons flour	1 tablespoon butter
1 recipe plain pastry	

Combine berries, rice syrup, flour, lemon juice and sea salt. Line pie pan with pastry, add filling, dot with butter and cover with top crust. Bake in very hot oven (450 degrees) for 10 minutes; reduce temperature to 350 degrees and bake 30 minutes longer.
Makes 1 9-inch pie.

✳

Fresh Pineapple Pie (Full of Life phase)

2 eggs	1 recipe plain pastry
1 1/3 cups rice syrup	1 tablespoon butter
2 cups shredded fresh pineapple	

Beat eggs slightly, add rice syrup, lemon juice and pineapple. Line pie pan with pastry, pour in filling, dot with butter and cover with top crust. Bake in very hot oven at 450 degrees for 10 minutes; reduce temperature to 350 degrees and bake 35 minutes longer or until pineapple is tender.
Makes 1 8-inch pie.

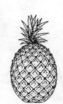

Cranberry Nut Cobbler

2 cups rice syrup
1 cup water
4 cups (1 Lb) cranberries
1 recipe Shortcake Biscuits*

1/2 cup chopped walnuts
2 tablespoons butter
grated rind of 1 orange

Heat syrup and water to boiling. Add cranberries, walnuts, orange rind and butter and let stand while mixing biscuit dough. Roll dough to 1/4 inch thickness. Fill individual baking dishes with cranberries and cover each with biscuit dough. Cut slits on top of dough to allow steam to escape. Bake in very hot oven at 450 degrees for 10 minutes, reduce heat to 350 degrees and bake 20 minutes longer.

*Makes 6 cobblers. (*listed below)*

Shortcake Biscuits

2 cups rice flour, sifted
3 teaspoons baking powder
4 tablespoons shortening

1/2 teaspoon sea salt
2 tablespoon rice syrup
3/4 cup goats milk

Sift dry ingredients together, add rice syrup and cut in shortening with 2 knives or pastry blender. Add goats milk, mix well and place on floured board. Knead lightly, pat out to 1/2 inch thickness and cut with round cutter. Place on greased baking sheet and chill until ready to bake. Bake in hot oven at 425 degrees for 20 minutes.

Makes 14 biscuits.

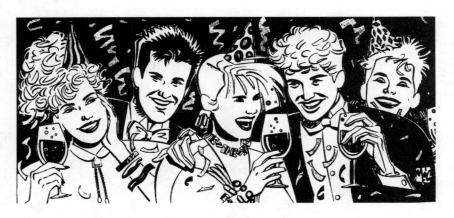

Conclusion

Before you start looking at the mouthwatering recipes, it is wise to reflect on the fact that "diets" never stay. But humans and their food-related problems do and in fact, increase as time goes on. A good food plan will not resolve all health problems. A broken heart, or hearing bad news, or ailments from a financial debacle will not be remedied by a food change. You will need homeopathic remedies for this. (See *"Human Condition: Critical)* But you should always try to eat sensible. When you are hurting the most, physically or emotionally, most of you have the tendency to go overboard with anything that even looks remotely like food. That this is detrimental to your state of mind and body is an understatement. It isn't easy when you are down to deprive yourself from your favorite dessert. But the feelings of guilt and depression and the hypoglycemic swings afterwards, are more difficult to handle. Be good to yourself when no one else seems to be. Open this book and look for a healthy, tasty alternative. Often, it will be the first step on the road to recovery!

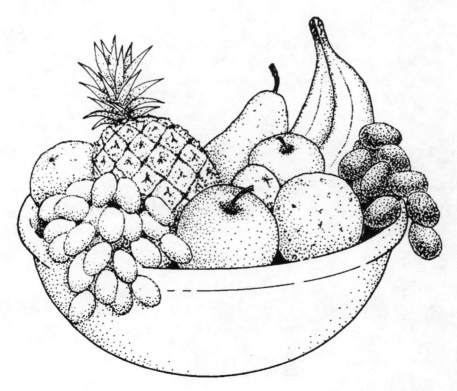

APPENDIX
Some Helpful Conversion Tables

OVEN TEMPERATURES

C	100	105	110	115	120	125	130	135	140	145	150	155	160	165
F	212	221	230	239	248	257	266	275	284	293	302	311	320	329

C	170	175	180	185	190	195	200	205	210	215	220	225	230	235
F	338	347	356	365	374	383	392	401	410	419	428	437	446	455

LIQUID MEASURES
(practical approximations)

1 cup	= 250 milliliters (ml)
	= 8 fluid ounces (fl. oz) USA
	= 8.7 fl oz Imperial (Australian old system)
	= 12 tablespoons
1 tablespoon	= 20 ml
	= 3/4 fl oz
	= 4 teaspoons
1 teaspoon	= 5 ml
	= 0.18 fl

FLOUR MEASURES
(practical approximations)

1 cup	= 140 grams (g)
	= 5 oz
	= 8 tablespoons
1 tablespoon	= 17 g
	= 1/2 oz
	= 4 teaspoons
1 teaspoon	= 4 g or 1/8 oz

GRAIN MEASURES
(practical approximations)

1 cup	= 190 g
	= 6.7 oz

INDEX

INDEX OF RECIPES

ORDERFORM

Please send (   ) copy(ies) of the book

"CANDIDA"
The Symptoms, the Causes, the Cure

Unit price: $10.00
Postage: $2.50
New Mexico residents add 6.25% sales tax

Ship to:

Name: _____

Street: _____

City: _____State:_____Zip:_____

Total purchase amount: $

Please send check or money order to:

Full of Life Publishing
500 N. Guadalupe St. G441
Santa Fe, New Mexico 87501

ORDERFORM

Please send ( ) copy(ies) of the book

"HUMAN CONDITION: *CRITICAL*"

Unit price: $12.95
Postage: $2.50
New Mexico residents add 6.25% sales tax

Ship to:

Name: _____

Street: _____

City: _____ State:_____ Zip:_____

Total purchase amount: $

Please send check or money order to:

Full of Life Publishing
500 N. Guadalupe St. G441
Santa Fe, New Mexico 87501

ORDERFORM

Please send (   ) copy(ies) of the book

"HOW TO DINE LIKE THE DEVIL AND FEEL
LIKE A SAINT"
Good-Bye To Guilty Eating

Unit price: $17.95
Postage: $2.50
New Mexico residents add 6.25% sales tax

Ship to:

Name: _____

Street: _____

City: _____ State: _____ Zip: _____

Total purchase amount: $

Please send check or money order to:

Full of Life Publishing
500 N. Guadalupe St. G441
Santa Fe, New Mexico 87501

ORDERFORM

Please send (   ) copy(ies) of the book

"FULL OF LIFE"
How to Achieve and Maintain Peak Immunity

Unit price: $12.95
Postage: $2.50
New Mexico residents add 6.25% sales tax

Ship to:

Name:_____

Street:_____

City:_____State:_____Zip:_____

Total purchase amount: $

Please send check or money order to:

Full of Life Publishing
500 N. Guadalupe St. G441
Santa Fe, New Mexico 87501